Easy Vegan Cookbook

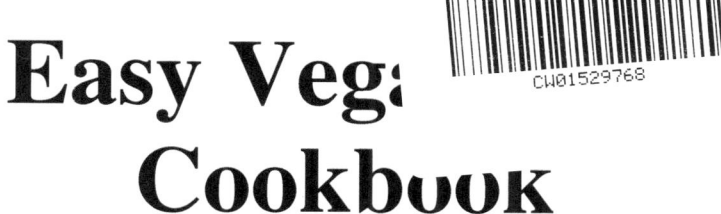

Delicious Recipes for Busy People

Shane Geraci

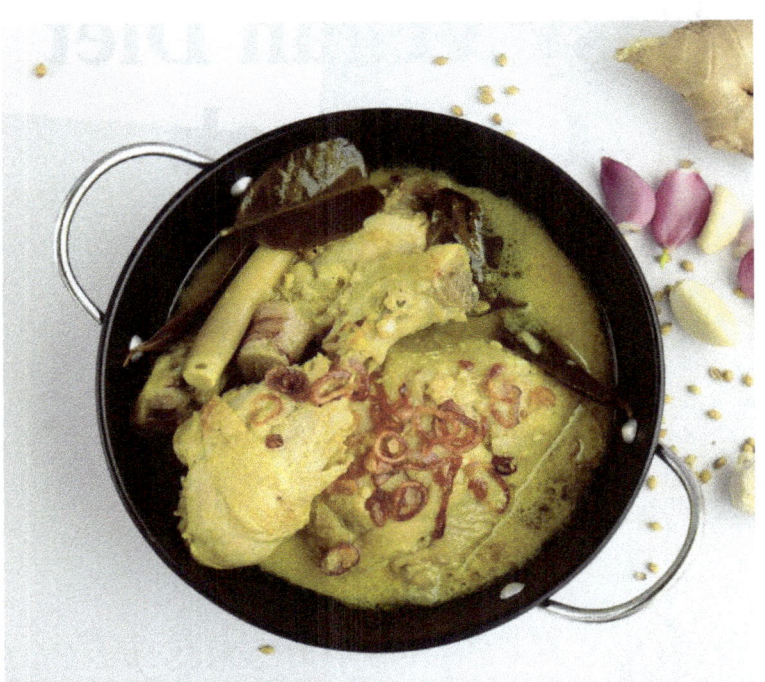

Easy Vegan Diet Cookbook

© Copyright 2021 by Shane Geraci - All rights reserved

Table of Contents

INTRODUCTION 1

MAIN FOODS 2

1. VEGAN LEMON COOKIES WITH CINNAMON AND CARROTS 3
2. POTATO AND SEITAN MEDALLIONS 5
3. BEETROOT HUMMUS 7
4. VEGAN COOKIES WITH ROSE PETALS 9
5. CREAM OF ZUCCHINI WITH SMOKED TEA 11
6. VEGAN MINI OMELETTE WITHOUT EGGS WITH VEGETABLES 13
7. MINI PLUMCAKE OF SOY MILK AND BITTER COCOA 15
8. MEATBALLS OF SEITAN, RAISINS AND ALMONDS 17
9. ORANGE RICE COOKIES 19
10. VEGAN PEA AND MINT MEATBALLS 21
11. FENNEL AND YOGURT CREAM 23
12. MILLET, CAROB AND BLUEBERRY BISCUITS 25
13. VEGAN PANNA COTTA WITH CHERRIES 27
14. AROMATIC SCONES 29
15. COFFEE, CHOCOLATE AND CARDAMOM MINI MUFFINS 31
16. SEITAN AND TURMERIC STEAK 33
17. SPICED MUFFINS 35
18. SOY YOGURT PLUMCAKE 37
19. TOFU MEDALLIONS 39
20. SEMOLINA FLOUR GNOCCHI WITH COURGETTES AND SAFFRON 41
21. SPOON SALAD 43
22. VEGAN BUCKWHEAT SCONES 45
23. VEGAN TEA COOKIES 47
24. VEGAN LASAGNA WITH SHIITAKE MUSHROOMS 49
25. VEGAN BANANA AND MATCHA TEA PLUMCAKE 51
26. SEITAN ESCALOPES WITH GRAPES 53
27. VEGAN GRATED CHEESE 55
28. VEGAN PUDDING WITH PEARS AND GOJI BERRIES 56
29. VEGAN SPREADABLE CHEESE 58
30. RISOTTO WITH BLUEBERRIES AND PORCINI MUSHROOMS 60
31. SPINACH AND TOFU ROLLS 62
32. VEGAN ALSATIAN APPLE PIE 64
33. LIME FLAVORED MUSHROOM CROUTONS 67

34.	ORANGE MUFFINS AND TONKA BEANS	69
35.	VEGAN LASAGNA WITH ESCAROLE, OLIVES AND WALNUTS	71
36.	VEGAN LASAGNA WITH BROCCOLI, WALNUTS AND SUNFLOWER SEEDS	73
37.	CREAM OF CARROTS AND PEANUT BUTTER WITH SPICED CROUTONS	76
38.	VEGAN LASAGNA WITH PUMPKIN AND TURNIP GREENS WITH OATMEAL BECHAMEL	78
39.	POLENTA VEGAN LASAGNA WITH RADICCHIO AND MUSHROOMS	81
40.	ORECCHIETTE WITH PEPPER CREAM	84
41.	VEGAN TART WITH TURMERIC CREAM	86
42.	ZUCCHINI WITH MANGO AND APPLES	88
43.	QUINOA VEGAN BURGER	90
44.	PUMPKIN, ROSEMARY, RAISINS AND CHOCOLATE MUFFINS	92
45.	PEAR AND CHOCOLATE VEGAN COOKIES	94
46.	WHOLEMEAL SHELLS WITH SAGE AND POTATOES	96
47.	MINT AND CHOCOLATE DONUTS	98
48.	WHOLEMEAL PUMPKIN PIE	100
49.	VEGAN PEAR, CHOCOLATE AND APPLE PIE	103
50.	VEGAN MUFFINS WITH ZUCCHINI AND DRIED TOMATOES	105

© Copyright 2021 by Shane Geraci - All rights reserved. The following Book is reproduced below with the goal of providing information that is as accurate and reliable as possible. Regardless, purchasing this Book can be seen as consent to the fact that both the publisher and the author of this book are in no way experts on the topics discussed within and that any recommendations or suggestions that are made herein are for entertainment purposes only. Professionals should be consulted as needed prior to undertaking any of the action endorsed herein.

This declaration is deemed fair and valid by both the American Bar Association and the Committee of Publishers Association and is legally binding throughout the United States.

Furthermore, the transmission, duplication, or reproduction of any of the following work including specific information will be considered an illegal act irrespective of if it is done electronically or in print. This extends to creating a secondary or tertiary copy of the work or a recorded copy and is only allowed with the express written consent from the Publisher. All additional right reserved.

The information in the following pages is broadly considered a truthful and accurate account of facts and as such, any inattention, use, or misuse of the information in question by the reader will render any resulting actions solely under their purview. There are no scenarios in which the publisher or the original author of this work can be in any fashion deemed liable for any hardship or damages that may befall them after undertaking information described herein.

Additionally, the information in the following pages is intended only for informational purposes and should thus be thought of as universal. As befitting its nature, it is presented without assurance regarding its prolonged validity or interim quality. Trademarks that are mentioned are done without written consent and can in no way be considered an endorsement from the trademark holder.

INTRODUCTION

You would think that because I've spent my career teaching people how to make plant-based meals, I'd be very passionate about cooking. The truth is, my favorite part about cooking is eating, and if I can make my meals with the least amount of time, effort, and dirty dishes, the food itself becomes even more enjoyable. Cook dried beans overnight while you sleep, add veggies and chili spices before you go to work, and when your day is done, you arrive toa a home filled with mouthwatering aromas and a comforting meal. It doesn't get much easier than that!

As you'll discover while reading Easy Vegan Diet Cookbook, gone are the days of using a 1970s-era burnt orange or avocado green Crock-Pot to figure out how you'll salvage inexpensive tough cuts of meat. Instead, spend the least amount of time in the kitchen while still serving flavorful, creative, nutritious meal for dinner Tl show you how to maximize your food budget and use your time in the kitchen efficiently by keeping all recipe prep times under 15 minutes, as well as give you some ideas for how to plan your weekly menus wisely.

The recipes in this book are designed for people like me who lave eating delicious things but don't love complicated cooking or doing massive amounts of dishes. These recipes are for busy people who want to feed themselves and their families nourishing food without spending a fortune, and who want focus on whole foods instead of packaged or processed.

Recipes

MAINS FOODS

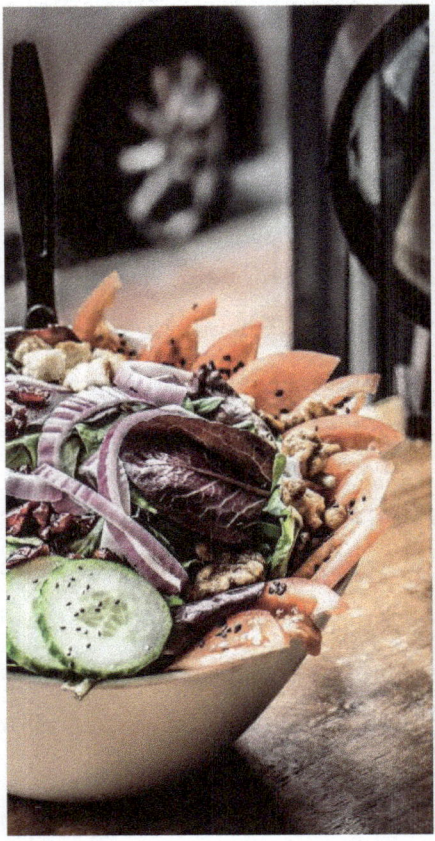
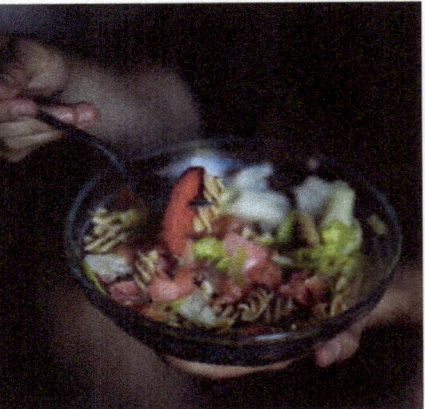
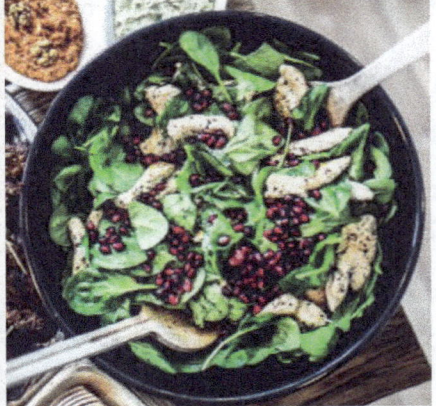

1. VEGAN LEMON COOKIES WITH CINNAMON AND CARROTS

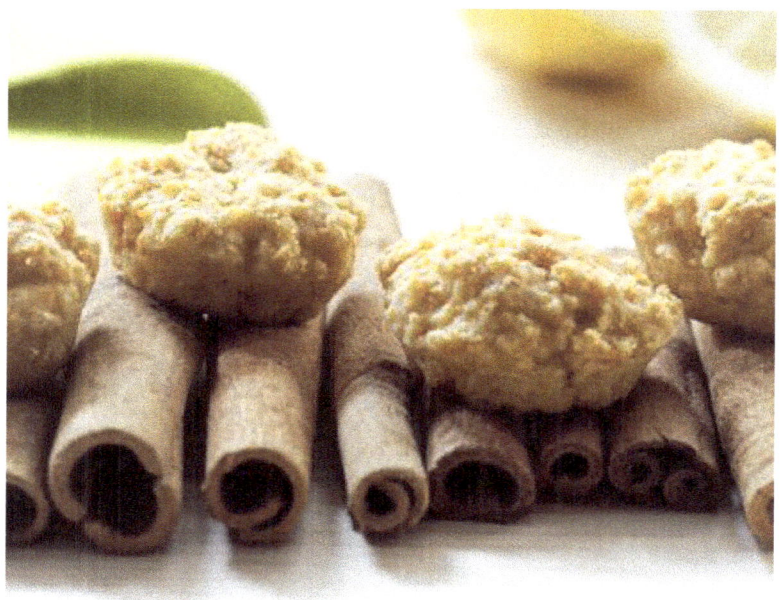

Ingredients

- 150 g of **corn meal** 's foil
- 75 g of **malt**
- 90 g of **carrots**
- 30 ml of corn oil
- 30 ml **of rice milk**
- 16 g of **natural yeast based on cream of tartar**
- the grated rind of one **lemon** (untreated)
- 1 teaspoon of **cinnamon**

- 1 pinch of salt

PREPARATION!

In a blender chop the peeled carrots and cut into small pieces with the salt, cinnamon and lemon zest until the mixture is well blended. Sift the flour together with the cream of tartar and add them to the freshly chopped mixture along with the rice milk, malt and oil. Mix the ingredients until you get a fairly soft dough: if lifted with a spoon, the dough should fall slowly.

We bake

Place the mixture in mini muffin molds (silicone ones are fine too) and bake at 190 ° C, static oven, for about 15 minutes: they must be golden brown. If you don't have the molds, you can also spoon the mixture onto a dripping pan covered with parchment paper, creating less regular and more rustic biscuits.

2. POTATO AND SEITAN MEDALLIONS

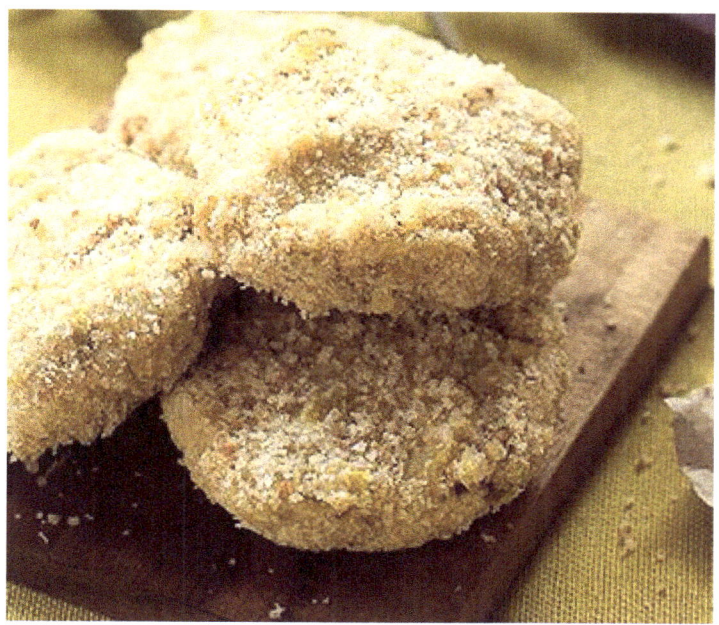

Ingredients

- 400 g of potatoes
- 100 g of **natural seitan**
- 1 **leek**
- breadcrumbs to taste
- extra virgin olive oil to taste
- salt and **pepper to** taste

PREPARATION!

The first step will be to peel the potatoes and cut them into coarsely cubes. Boil them in a fairly large pot, in plenty of salted water, until you can pierce them with a wooden toothpick. Separately, peel the leek and pour it into the food processor together with the seitan: both ingredients must be finely chopped, so as to be well workable.

Now heat a drizzle of oil in a pan and add the chopped leek and seitan. Cook for a few minutes and at the end add the potatoes, which you will mash with a fork, salt and pepper according to your taste. You will have to be careful to mix the ingredients well, then let them cool.

We form the medallions

With slightly moist hands, form morsels or medallions of the size you like best (the important thing is that they all have the same size, so as to cook evenly), pass them in breadcrumbs and place them in the dripping pan that you will have lined with baking paper. . Bake at 180 ° C for about 10 minutes, being careful to turn the medallions halfway through cooking.

3. BEETROOT HUMMUS

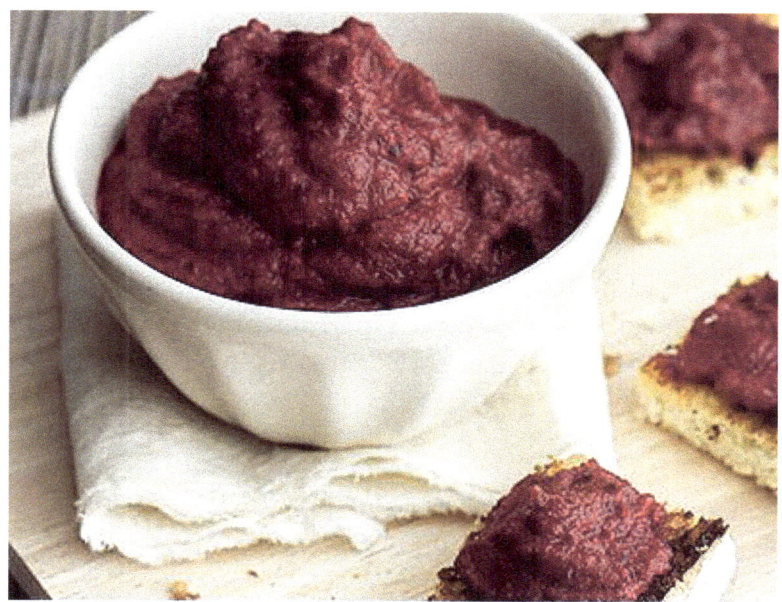

Ingredients

- 400 g of precooked beetroot
- 230 g of **chickpeas** cooked
  (or 1 equ one of **chickpeas** drained)
- 2 tablespoons of Arame **tahini** sauce
- 1 **lemon**
- 1 pinch of salt
- 1 teaspoon of **cumin**
- extra virgin olive oil

PREPARATION!

We blend the ingredients

Preparing beet hummus is very quick and easy. In your food processor, pour the ingredients, then the chickpeas, beetroot, tahini, salt, lemon juice and cumin. Blend until you get a homogeneous cream and, if necessary, add a little oil or a drop of water to soften everything.

We serve

Hummus is an ideal cream to spread on croutons; in particular, this variant of the traditional cream has a more intense flavor, given by the tahina, a paste of toasted sesame seeds, flavored with arame seaweed.

4. VEGAN COOKIES WITH ROSE PETALS

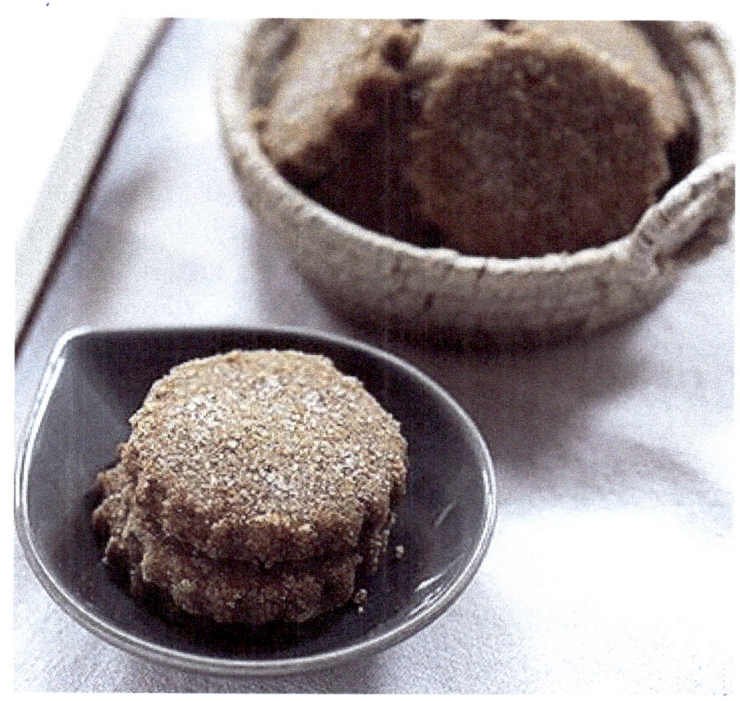

Ingredients

- 100 g of whole meal flour
- 100 g of **rice flour**
- 1 teaspoon of **cream** of **tartar**
- 80g brown sugar + for sprinkling
- 2 teaspoons of **malt**
- 120 ml of sunflower or corn oil
- Crumbled dried rose petals

PREPARATION!

The dough
In a large bowl or on a wooden pastry board, sift the two flours together, add the yeast, the brown sugar, the two teaspoons of malt, the crumbled rose petals (available in herbal medicine) and add, to thread, oil, starting to mix. Continue until you get a ball of dough: don't be scared if the dough is particularly soft. Wrap the ball of dough in cling film and let it rest in the refrigerator for at least 2 hours.

Let's work it
After the two hours have passed, the dough will not be hard, as happens with the classic short crust pastry, but always soft, but workable. Lean on a wooden pastry board, lightly flour it and with the help of a floured rolling pin, proceed by rolling out the dough. If it breaks, don't worry, fix any "leaks" and proceed. Roll out the mixture to obtain a surface of about 2 cm thick, cut the shapes of the biscuits. Sprinkle each biscuit with a pinch of brown sugar.

Bake
on a baking tray covered with parchment paper, lying biscuits (help with a spoon or a spatula if they were to be too soft) and cook in a pre-heated oven at 180 ° C for about 10 minutes.

5. CREAM OF ZUCCHINI WITH SMOKED TEA

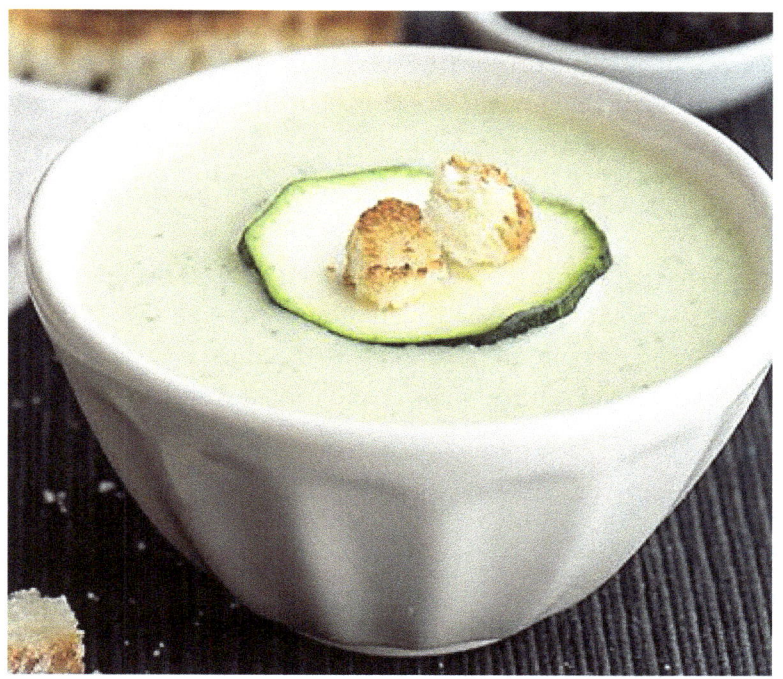

Ingredients

- 400 g of **zucchini**
- 180 g of velvety **tofu**
- 1 **leek**
- 600 ml of smoked tea
- extra virgin olive oil
- salt and **pepper to** taste

PREPARATION!

PREPARATION the zucchini

Clean the leek and slice it into slices and then let it dry for a few minutes in a pan with a drizzle of extra virgin olive oil. Now add the courgettes, which you have previously washed and coarsely chopped, and cook for a few minutes.

We whisk

Now pour in the broth flavored with smoked tea and bring to a boil, continuing to cook for another 15/20 minutes. At the end of cooking, add the tofu and with an immersion blender reduce everything to a creamy mixture. Add salt and pepper and serve lukewarm.

6. VEGAN MINI OMELETTE WITHOUT EGGS WITH VEGETABLES

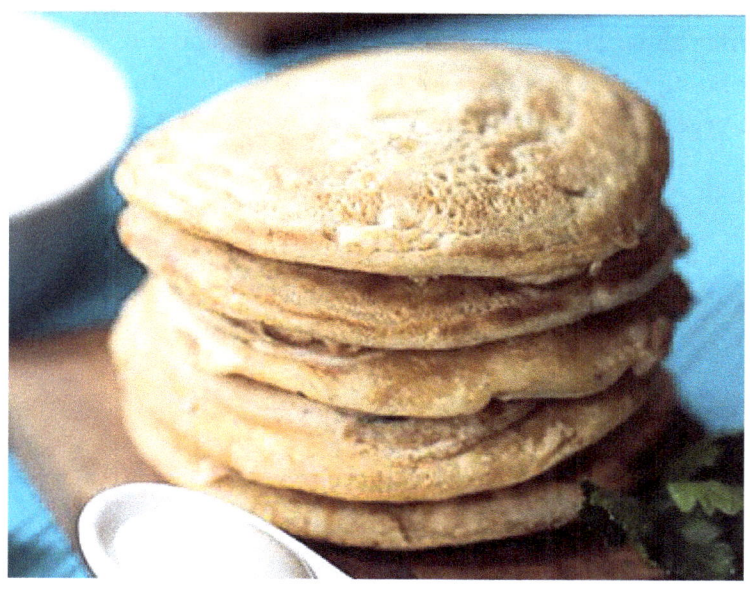

Ingredients

- 150 ml **of soy milk**
- 50 g of **flour**
- 50 g of **chickpea flour** or **corn flour** foil
- 1 grated **courgette**
- 2 grated **carrots**
- extra virgin olive oil
- 1/2 teaspoon of baking soda
- 1 level teaspoon of curry
- Salt to taste

PREPARATION!

In a large bowl, mix the sifted flours with the milk, add the salt, curry and baking soda. Then add the grated vegetables and mix gently, incorporating the elements well into the mixture. Of course, you can use the vegetables you prefer.

In the pan

In a non-stick pan, heat a tablespoon of olive oil, then with a spoon or ladle equipped with a spout pour small quantities of mixture into the pan, cook first on one side and then on the other using a spatula to turn the omelettes . Cooking must take place over a moderate heat and will be optimal when both sides have a golden and not burnt color.

You can also make an omelet **without eggs** big instead of 10 small.

7. MINI PLUMCAKE OF SOY MILK AND BITTER COCOA

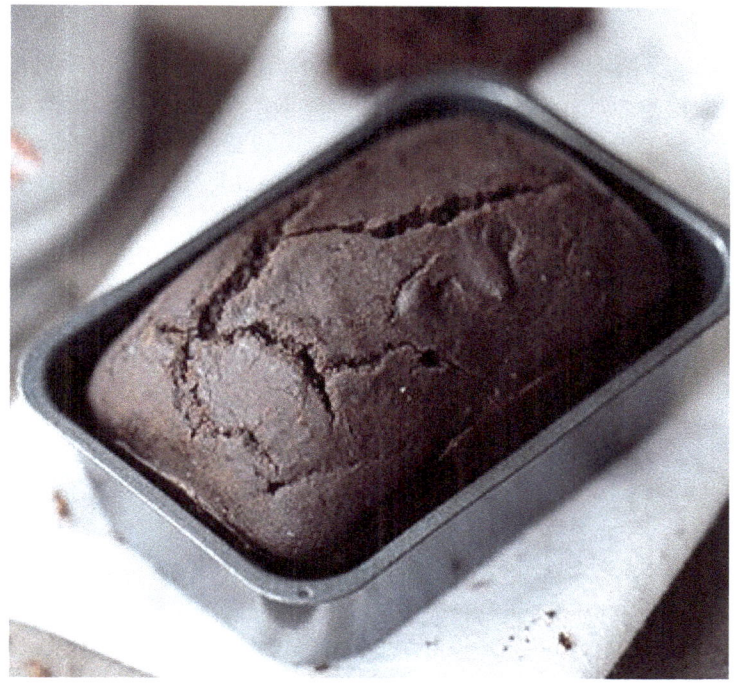

Ingredients

- 130 g of flour 0 or wholemeal flour
- 70 g of brown sugar
- 150 ml **of soy milk**
- 2 tablespoons of corn oil
- 4 g of **cream** of **tartar**
- 40 g of unsweetened cocoa powder

PREPARATION!

The dough

In a large bowl sift the 0 flour together with the baking powder, then add the granulated sugar (you can also replace it with corn malt syrup, even if the result will be decidedly more bitter due to the cocoa) and then to follow the cocoa powder.: mix the powders well together.

Liquids

Now add the liquids: corn oil and soy milk (you can replace it with rice milk if you prefer this flavor: to find out more). Mix the mixture with the help of a spoon until it is very homogeneous: it must not be excessively solid / lumpy.

We bake

Pour the mixture into molds (you can also use muffin molds) and bake in a preheated static oven at 180 ° C for about 15/20 minutes. Once ready, let the cakes cool (preferably on a wire rack) and serve them.

8. MEATBALLS OF SEITAN, RAISINS AND ALMONDS

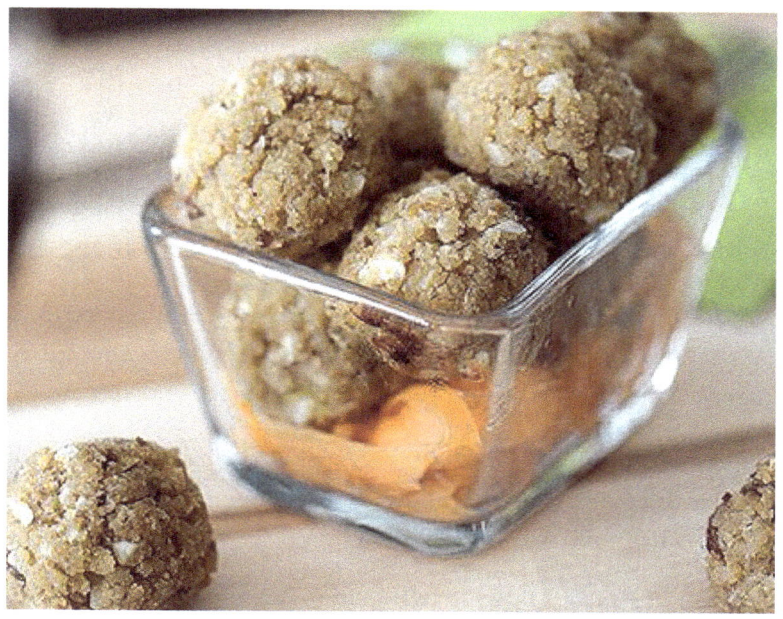

Ingredients

- 300 g of **seitan**
- 2 tablespoons **of chickpea flour**
- 50 g of **raisins**
- 50 g of **almonds**
- 1/2 **leek**
- extra virgin olive oil to taste
- salt and **pepper to** taste

Tools

- **hand blender** or **food processor**
- baking **tray**

PREPARATION!

First, let the raisins soak in warm water for a few minutes. Meanwhile, in a large non-stick pan, toast the almonds which you will then finely chop once cooled. The toasting is used to give a stronger flavor to your meatballs.

In a pan, heat a drizzle of oil and stew the leek that you have cut into slices. As soon as it takes a little color, add the seitan cut into cubes and the squeezed raisins. Sauté for a few minutes, just to add flavor.

Then pour everything into a food processor and chop very finely. The mixture must become quite sticky, to then be able to work it with your hands. In a bowl, mix all the ingredients, also adding the almonds and chickpea flour.

With slightly damp hands, form small balls with a diameter of about 1.5 centimeters and place them in the baking tray lined with baking paper. Cook at 180 ° C for about 10 minutes, being careful to turn them halfway through cooking.

9. **ORANGE RICE COOKIES**

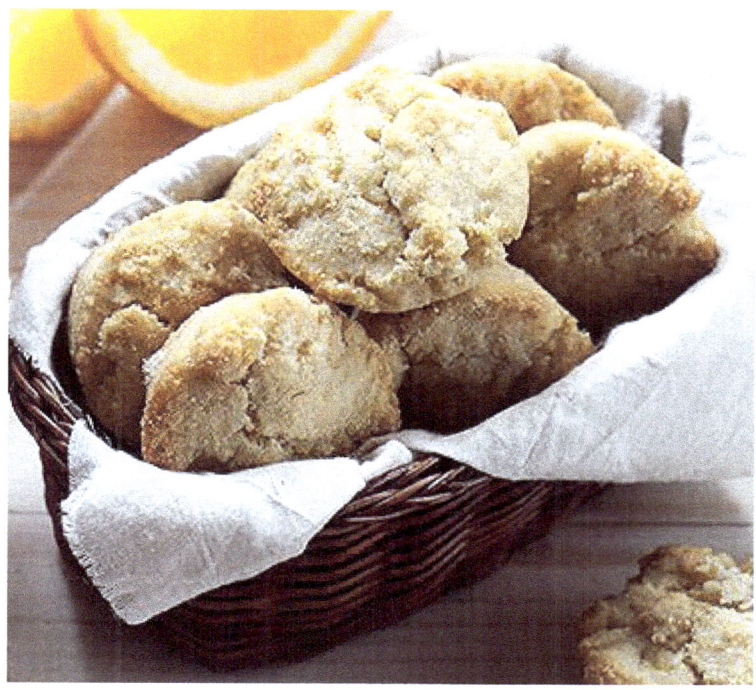

Ingredients

- 250 g of **rice flour**
- 75 g of **millet** flour
- 100 g of **rice milk**
- 100 g of **rice malt**
- 90 g of corn oil
- 10 g of olive oil
- zest and juice of an **orange**
- 1 sachet of **cream** of **tartar**

- a pinch of salt

PREPARATION!

The dough: the flours

In a bowl sift the two flours in order to avoid lumps and add the other dry ingredients, that is cream of tartar, salt and orange peel (better if organic, especially when we want to use the peel of citrus fruits).

Liquids

In another container, however, dissolve the malt with the liquids: if you want you can help yourself with an electric whisk or an immersion blender to mix everything well.

We bake

Now add the dry ingredients to the liquid ones and mix them vigorously until you get a uniform, not too liquid mixture. You can use a pastry bag to create special shapes for your biscuits with the dough or pour the dough into mini molds.

You will go to bake in a preheated static oven at 190 ° C for about 15 minutes, the rice biscuits should be slightly browned on the surface.

10. VEGAN PEA AND MINT MEATBALLS

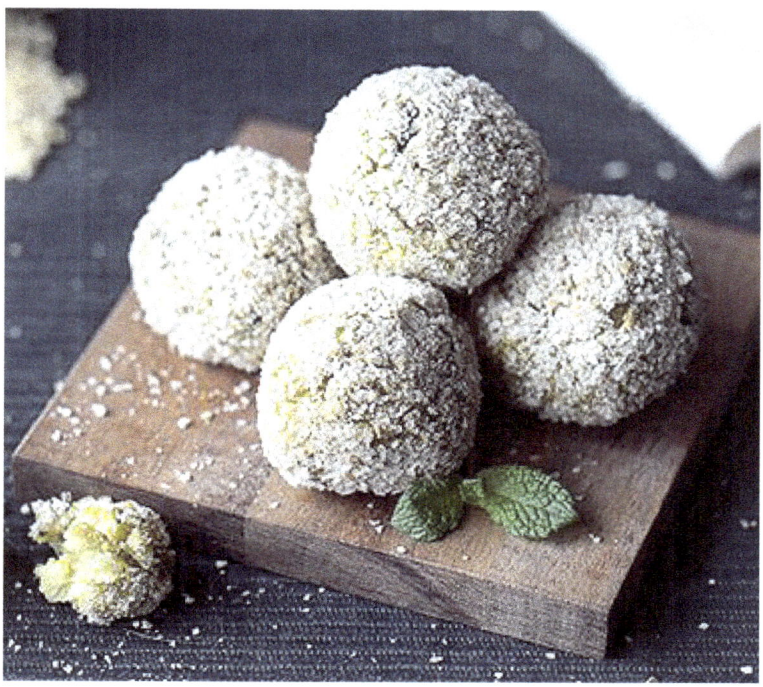

Ingredients

- 400 g of boiled **peas**
- 100 g of **millet**
- 1 shallot
- 6 fresh mint leaves
- breadcrumbs to taste
- 50 g of **tofu** soft (optional)
- salt and **pepper to** taste

PREPARATION!

PREPARATION the millet

First, blend the peas in a food processor together with the shallot and mint. Separately, in a saucepan, cook the millet in 300 ml of water (the millet-water ratio is always 1 to 3). Cooking will take place by absorption: that is, you will have to wait for the millet to have absorbed all the liquid, only then will it be ready to be used.

Let's mix the ingredients ...

Mix by blending the pea cream with the soft tofu and the millet you just cooked, adding as much breadcrumbs as you need to obtain a hand-workable mixture.

... And we form the meatballs

Season with salt and pepper and, with the help of a spoon, form meatballs. At the end of the operation, pass each meatball in breadcrumbs or in a bit of re-milled durum wheat semolina flour. This will provide the meatballs with a nice golden color and just the right crunchiness.

In the oven

Bake the pea and mint meatballs on a baking tray covered with parchment paper at 180 degrees (static oven) for a few minutes, until golden on the surface.

11. FENNEL AND YOGURT CREAM

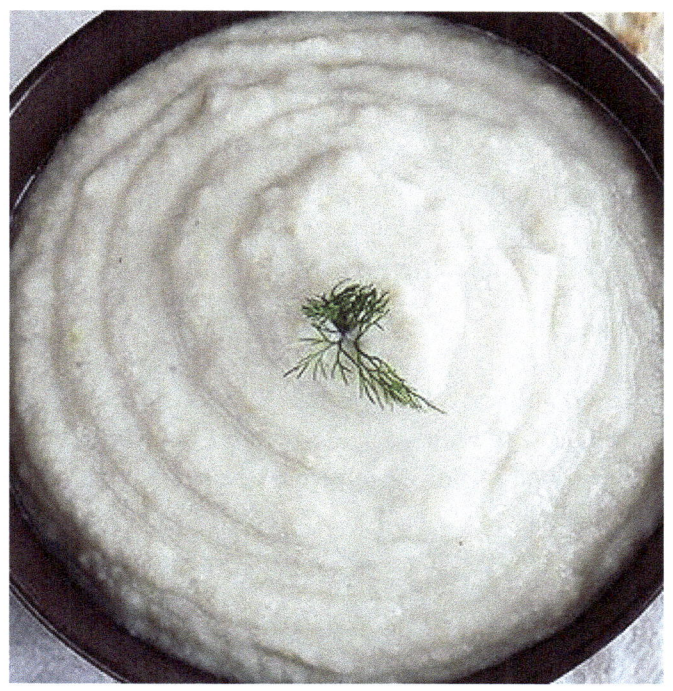

Ingredients

- 300 g of **fennel**
- 300 g of boiled potatoes
- 500 ml of **vegetable broth**
- 1 **leek**
- 250 g unsweetened soy yogurt
- extra virgin olive oil to taste
- salt and **pepper to** taste

PREPARATION!

Let's cook the fennel

First, clean the fennel and cut it very finely. Separately, in a non-stick pan, stew the leek cut into slices in a drizzle of extra virgin olive oil. Now add the chopped fennel, cook for a few minutes and pour the vegetable broth. Cook, stirring occasionally, for about 20 minutes, after which the vegetables should be very soft.

We prepare the cream

Now pour everything into a large container, add the boiled and diced potatoes and blend with an immersion blender. Add salt and pepper to flavor your cream and to finish the yogurt, which you will mix well with the other ingredients.

As soon as the mixture becomes homogeneous, it will be ready to be served.

12. MILLET, CAROB AND BLUEBERRY BISCUITS

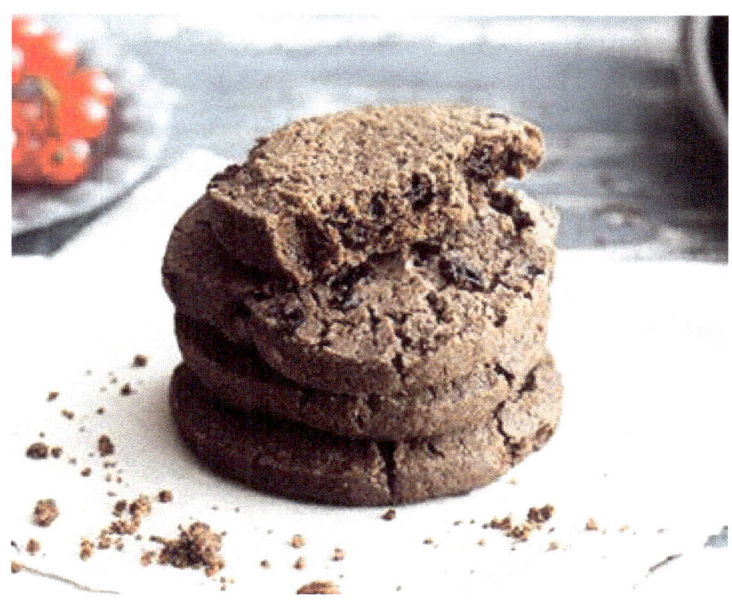

Ingredients

150 g of flour of **a mile** (or 75 g of **rice flour** and 75 g of flour of **millet**)
25 g of flour 0
50 g of flour of **carob**
50 g of **corn starch** (cornstarch)
1 pinch of salt
50 g of **rice** (or soy) **milk**
140 g of soy butter
140 g of cane sugar
50 g dried blueberries

PREPARATION!

The dough

In a planetary mixer (or by hand with a whisk) whip the soy butter with the sugar until you get a soft and fluffy cream. Separately, in a large bowl, sift all the flours and add the dose of starch and a pinch of salt. Then add the butter worked with the sugar, the powders and the rice milk: now mix all the ingredients well. Finally, add the blueberries and continue to mix. You can replace the blueberries with currants or other red fruits to taste, or to make everything even more "chocolaty" put some chocolate chips.

Let's shape the cookies!

With the mixture obtained try to form a sort of cylinder, perhaps with the help of baking paper. Cover it with cling film (or with the parchment paper just used) and put everything in the freezer for about 1 hour and until it is very compact. Slice the cylinder with the help of a sharp knife with a smooth blade, trying to obtain discs about 1 cm thick which you will then place on a baking tray covered with baking paper.

Let's bake!

Bake in a static oven at 180 degrees for about 15/20 minutes. Before serving, let it cool

13. VEGAN PANNA COTTA WITH CHERRIES

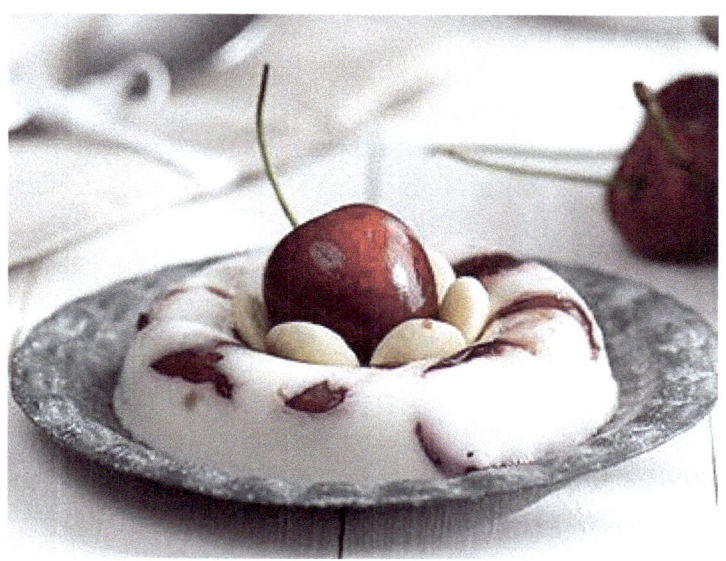

Ingredients

- 500 ml **of soy cream**
- 80 g of whole cane sugar
- 1 berry **vanilla**
- 1 teaspoon of **agar** (about 4 g)
- 20 **cherries** + 4 to decorate
- 60 g of **almonds**
- **soy** or rice **milk** to dissolve the **agar**

PREPARATION!

We prepare the fruit

First remove the stones from the cherries and wash them well under running water. In a saucepan, cook them over low heat with a drizzle of water and 2 tablespoons of whole brown sugar until they become slightly soft. Quickly toast the coarsely chopped almonds in the oven or in a non-stick pan, keeping a few aside to decorate the cake.

We heat the soy cream

In a saucepan, heat the vegetable cream, pour the sugar and the seeds of the vanilla bean. Bring to a light boil and add the seaweed agar agar, which you have previously dissolved in a drop of soy or rice milk at room temperature.

We put in the molds

Take some cocottine or small glass cups and place the cooked cherries on the base, cover with cream and decorate with almonds. Let it rest in the fridge for about 2 hours. Once firm, the panna cotta is ready to be served: decorate it with a fresh cherry and chopped almonds.

14. **AROMATIC SCONES**

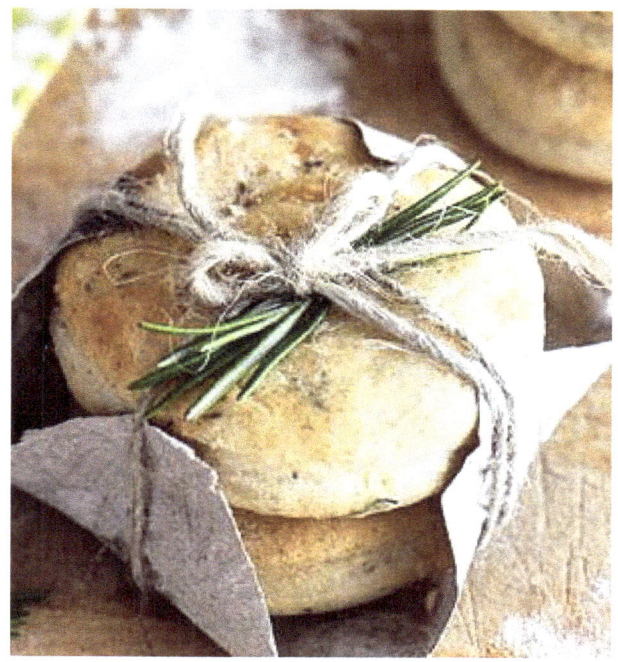

Ingredients

- 300 g of flour 00
- 150 g of warm water
- 10 g of fresh brewer's yeast
- mixed Provencal herbs (dried or fresh)
- 3 g of granulated sugar
- 9 g of fine salt
- 15 g of extra virgin olive oil

PREPARATION!

The dough

First, dissolve the fresh yeast and sugar in the warm water. Separately, in a large bowl, combine the sifted flour, salt, herbs and oil. Proceed by kneading vigorously (preferably on a porous surface such as wood) until you get a smooth and homogeneous dough. Let the dough rise for about 30 minutes: the temperature should be slightly higher than the room temperature. We therefore recommend that you place the dough in the oven that is turned off, but with the light on and covered with a clean, slightly moistened cloth. Meanwhile, in a small bowl, make an emulsion with oil and water.

The second leavening

After the first leavening time, roll out the dough with a rolling pin to a thickness of about 1 cm and cut it out with round pastry cups: place the disks obtained in a pan covered with lightly greased baking paper. Before baking, brush the scones with the emulsion: you will have to let them rise again for about 30 minutes, always in a warm place and away from drafts.

Let's bake!

After 30 minutes, sprinkle with coarse salt and mix at 200 degrees for about 20/25 minutes. During cooking, place a bowl with water in order to maintain controlled humidity in the oven. Once out of the oven, let the scones cool on a wire rack (not on the dripping pan) and you will be ready to enjoy them.

15. COFFEE, CHOCOLATE AND CARDAMOM MINI MUFFINS

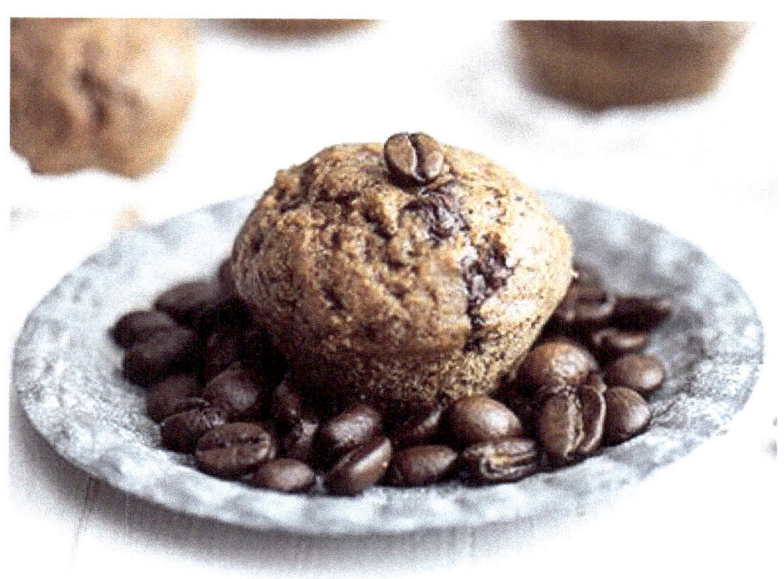

Ingredients

- 200 g of **whole meal flour**
- 50 ml of corn oil
- 50 ml of **coffee** (a **coffee pot** of 2)
- 100 ml of **soy milk** (or other vegetable milk to taste)
- 1 teaspoon of **coffee** powder
- 50 g of **hazelnuts**
- 1/2 sachet of baking powder

- 2 - 3 **cardamom** pods
- 2 teaspoons of cocoa powder
- 50 g of brown sugar
- dark chocolate chips to taste

PREPARATION!

Let's prepare the coffee

First make the coffee with the mocha: once ready, infuse the cardamom pods, after having crushed them well in a pestle or with the blade of a knife. Leave everything to rest while you prepare the rest of the dough. Aside, coarsely chop the hazelnuts.

Let's make muffins

In a large bowl put the sifted flour with baking powder, sugar, coffee powder, cocoa. Add the seed oil, the milk at room temperature, and then the coffee, taking care before filtering it to prevent the remains of the cardamom berries from ending up in the dough. Start mixing everything well and, at the end, add the chocolate chips and the chopped hazelnuts. The dough will be quite soft.

Ready for the oven!

Turn on the oven to 180 ° C and start putting the mixture into the molds with the help of two spoons: do not exceed 3/4 of each mold. Once finished, put the molds in the oven for 15 minutes. You just have to wait for the cooking and then ... devour the sweets!

16. SEITAN AND TURMERIC STEAK

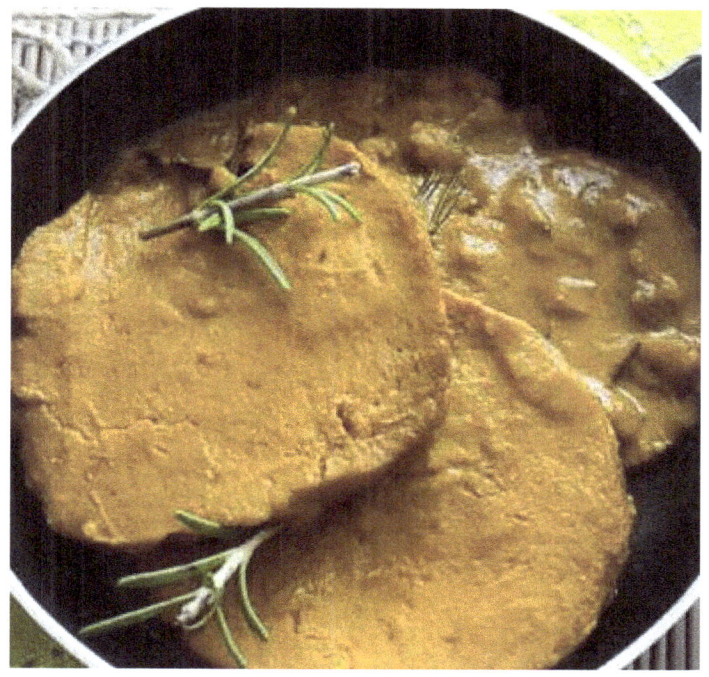

Ingredients

- 300 g of **seitan** medallions
- 1 onion
- 3 - 4 teaspoons of **turmeric**
- white wine to taste
- 2 - 3 sprigs of **rosemary**
- Salt to taste
- olive oil

PREPARATION!

First we stew the onion ...

First, simmer the finely chopped onion with a drizzle of oil, a drop of water and a pinch of salt in a fairly large non-stick pan. Meanwhile, cut the medallions in half lengthwise, so that you get two steaks from each.

Now let's put the seitan

When the onion is stewed, add the seitan and brown it, turning it with the help of a fork, for a couple of minutes. Now sprinkle the turmeric on the medallions, add the sprigs of rosemary and cover everything with plenty of white wine. Cook with the lid on over medium-low heat. From time to time, check that the liquid has not been completely absorbed: the seitan steaks will be ready when a homogeneous cream has formed.

17. **SPICED MUFFINS**

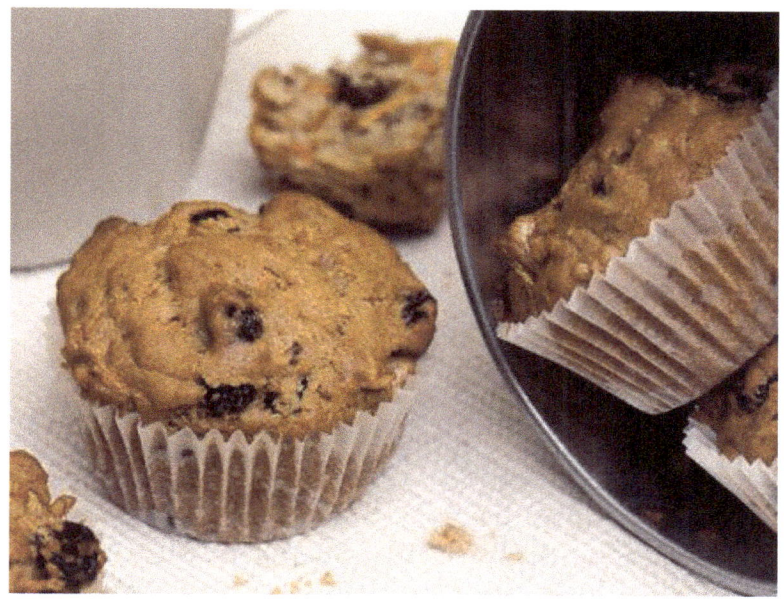

Ingredients

- 300 g of flour 0
- 1 pinch of salt
- 1 sachet of **cream** of **tartar**
- 1 teaspoon of **cinnamon**
- 50 ml of **apple** juice
- 120 g of **maple** or agave **syrup**
- 120 g of corn oil
- 100 g of **carrots**
- 100 g of **raisins**

- 100 g of **walnuts**

PREPARATION!

Let's prepare the muffin dough

In a large bowl, mix the dry ingredients together: then add the sifted flour (to avoid lumps), the teaspoon of cinnamon, a pinch of salt and the cream of tartar. In another bowl, put the liquid ingredients, then the oil, apple juice and maple syrup (or alternatively that of agave).

Carrots, raisins and nuts

Meanwhile, soak the raisins in a little warm water so that it regains its soft and sugary consistency. Separately, peel the carrots and cut them into julienne strips (if you want you can also cut them into thin strips and then into small cubes, but really small to avoid problems in cooking). Separately, roughly cut the walnut kernels with a knife.

Let's mix and bake!

Now it's time to combine all the ingredients: take the liquids, add them to the powders and start mixing. Once you have a homogeneous mixture, add the squeezed raisins, chopped walnuts and carrots. Mix well. If the dough is too dry, you can add a drop of apple juice.

Take your muffin pan and, with the help of a spoon, pour the mixture directly into the pan or into the cups, if you use them. You will have to bake the muffins for about 45-50 minutes in a static oven at 180 ° and then… enjoy your meal!

18. SOY YOGURT PLUMCAKE

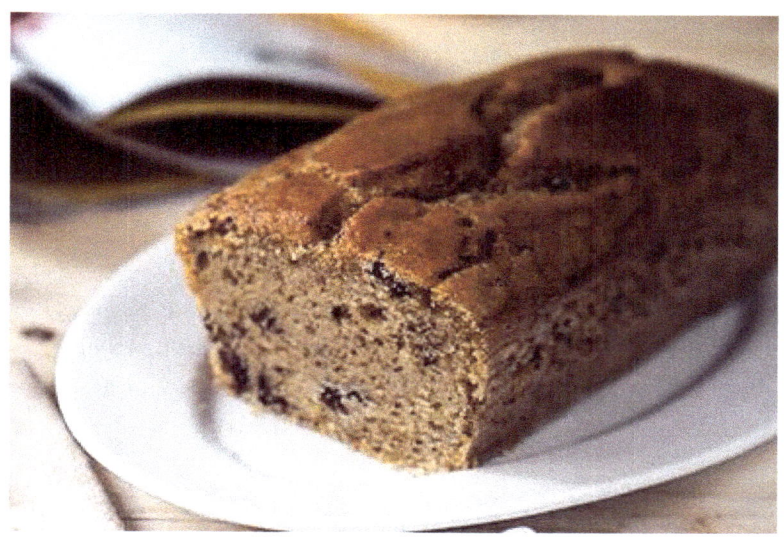

Ingredients

- 250 g of soy yogurt
- 250 g type 2 flour (semi wholemeal)
- 50 g of **cornstarch**
- 50 g of dark chocolate
- 130 g of **oat** milk
- 80 g of corn oil
- 120 g of brown sugar
- 1 sachet of **cream** of **tartar**
- zest of 1 **orange**
- a pinch of salt

PREPARATION!

Let's mix the liquids first

In a blender, pour the sugar and chop it to make it as fine as possible; add the yogurt, then the oil, milk and a pinch of salt. Always emulsify everything with the blender.

And now the powders

Separately, sift the flour, cornstarch and cream of tartar in a large bowl. Add the grated orange zest and the coarsely chopped chocolate with a knife. You can also replace the chocolate with **cocoa bean** grains (you can find it in organic food stores)

We mix and bake

Then add the liquids to the dry ingredients and mix with a spoon until the mixture is smooth and homogeneous. Now pour the mixture into a previously oiled and floured plumcake mold; cook in a static oven for about 35 minutes at 180 degrees. As always, use a wooden toothpick to check the cooking well before turning off the oven.

19. TOFU MEDALLIONS

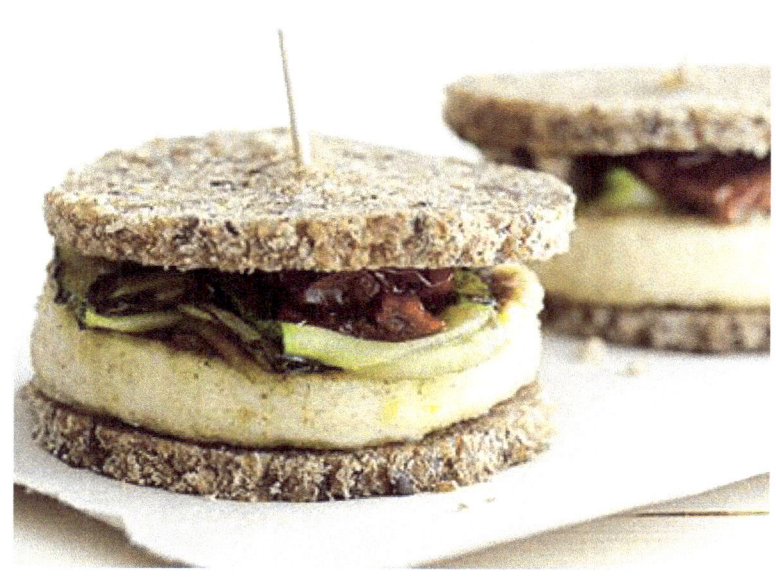

Ingredients

8 dried **tomatoes in** oil
1 large **courgette**
1 red onion
1 stick of **tofu**
8 slices of bread or small rolls
salt to taste
rice flour to taste (alternatively wholemeal flour)
extra virgin olive oil to taste

PREPARATION!

Let's prepare the tofu

With a pasta bowl cut both the bread, which you can then go to toast, and the tofu in order to have medallions of equal size. Blanch the latter in water to remove some of that bitter taste that characterizes it, a couple of minutes will be enough. Dip the tofu in the rice flour (or wholemeal if you prefer) and cook it lightly in a non-stick pan with a drizzle of hot oil for a few minutes on each side.

Go with the vegetables

Cut the onion into rings and fry it with a little olive oil while the courgettis cut them lengthwise into very thin slices (help yourself if you are more comfortable with a potato peeler) and blanch them on a hot plate. Salt them lightly. Take the dried tomatoes and let them drain well from the excess oil.

Ready medallions!

When all the ingredients are cooked, take a medallion of toasted bread, place the tofu, the onion slices, the courgettis and finally the dried tomatoes on it. Close with a last layer of bread and stop everything with toothpicks, perhaps cocktail ones, to make your dish even more beautiful to bring to the table!

20. SEMOLINA FLOUR GNOCCHI WITH COURGETTES AND SAFFRON

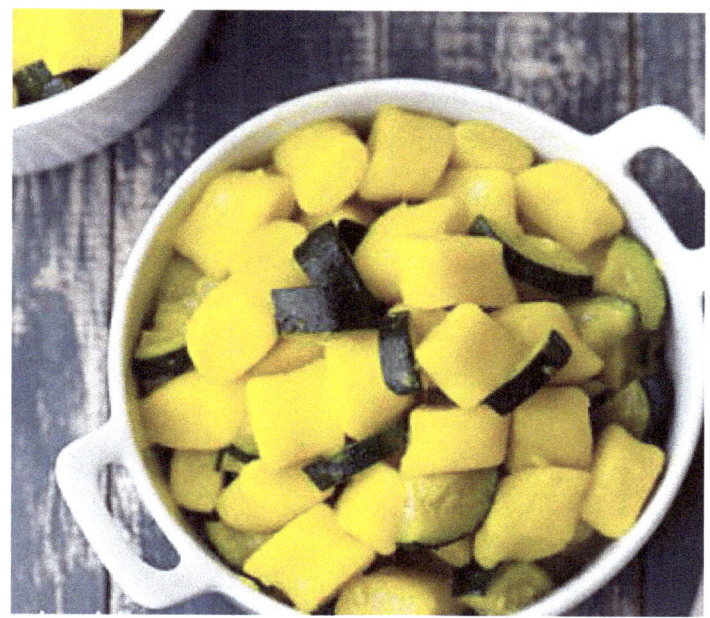

Ingredients

- 500 g durum wheat semolina flour (also re-milled will do)
- 250 ml of hot water
- 10 g of salt

For the dressing

- 1/2 onion
- 6 small **courgettes**
- salt
- extra virgin olive oil
- 1 sachet of saffron

PREPARATION!

How to prepare the pasta

To prepare the dumplings it is necessary to arrange the flour in a fountain and gradually add the water in the center. Slowly from the outside, mix a little flour with the water and continue until all the liquid has been completely absorbed. At this point the flour will have a consistency that can be worked with your hands. It will continue to work until it is completely smooth and homogeneous. It will take about 15 minutes of processing. With your hands, form a dough and wrap it in cling film: let it rest for about half an hour at room temperature.

And now the dumplings

At the end of the rest period, take the dough into small pieces and form sticks (such as bread sticks) with a diameter of 1 centimeter and cut them into cylinders, always about 1 centimeter in length. You will go there as they are ready to place in a bowl or tray with a little flour to prevent them from sticking together. While preparing the dumplings, remember to always keep the dough covered to prevent it from drying out excessively. Bring the salted water to a boil in a saucepan and cook the pasta for about 15 minutes.

The dressing with zucchini and saffron

While the pasta is cooking, cut the onion into strips and sauté it in a pan with a drizzle of oil. Add the courgettes that you have peeled and cut into small cubes. Season with salt and cook until the vegetables are well cooked but still crunchy. Once the pasta is cooked, drain it and set aside a little cooking liquid and add it to the pan with the vegetables. Add the saffron dissolved in the cooking water. Stir and serve.

You can add some black pepper or thyme to give the recipe an extra touch!

21. SPOON SALAD

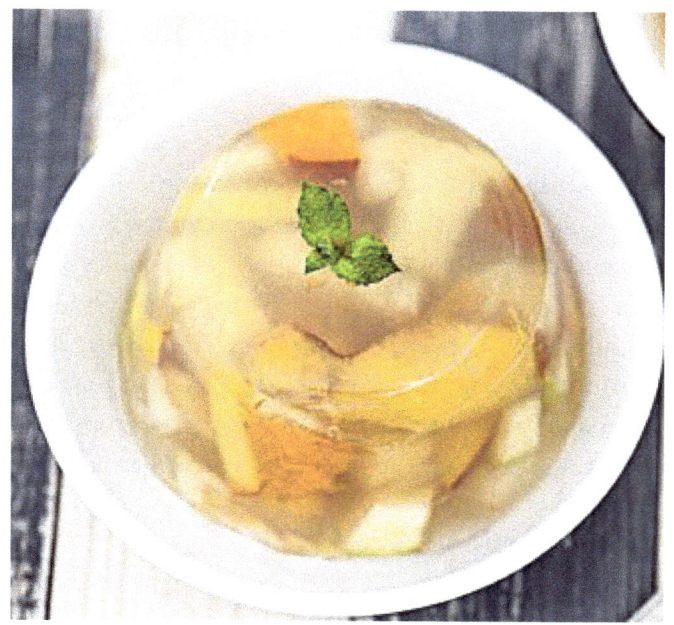

Ingredients

- 2 **apricots**
- 1 walnut peach
- 1 pear
- 1 **apple**
- 500 ml of **apple** juice
- 1 teaspoon of powdered **agar agar** (about 4 grams)
- mint leaves or red fruits to decorate

PREPARATION!

We prepare the jelly

First, dissolve the agar agar in a little cold water. In a saucepan, bring the apple juice to a light boil and add the dissolved agar agar while continuing to simmer the juice for about 1 minute, then turn off and let it cool.

We cut the fruit

Apart, wash the fruit; pitted apricots and peaches, cored apple and pear. If the fruit is organic, keep the peel, a source of vitamins. Now cut the fruit into cubes and distribute it evenly in 4 bowls and also pour the apple juice with the agar agar. Put the cups in the fridge for about 2 hours, once the cooling time has elapsed, remove them from the fridge, turn them over and turn them out with a slight pressure. If you find it difficult to extract the cake from the mold, dip the base of the cups in two fingers of boiling water and repeat the operation. Serve garnished with mint leaves and red fruits.

22. **VEGAN BUCKWHEAT SCONES**

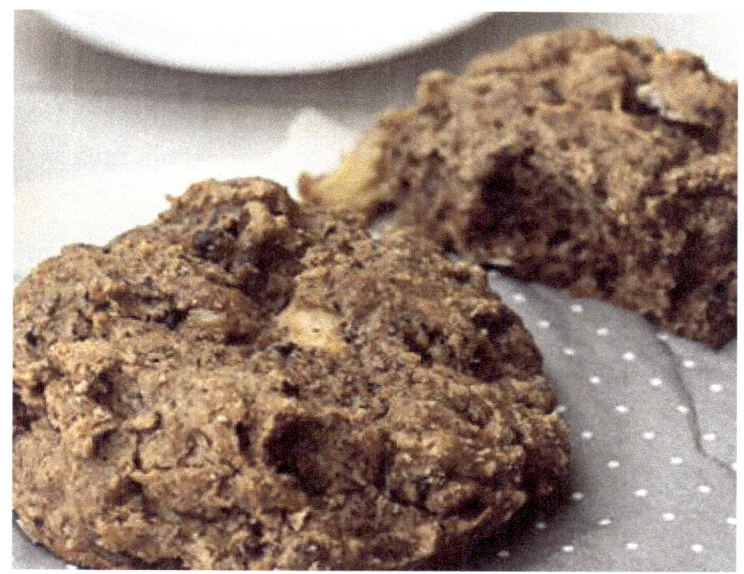

Ingredients

- 250 g of **buckwheat** flour
- 70 g of **almond flour**
- 2 **apples**
- 150 g of **almond milk**
- 100 g of brown sugar
- 1 sachet of yeast (16g)
- 1 teaspoon of **cinnamon**
- 1 teaspoon of baking soda
- 1 pinch of salt

PREPARATION!

Cut the apples into cubes without their peel. Separately, sift the flour and baking powder and add all the other dry ingredients. Add the apples and, little by little, the milk. The dough you will get should not be too sticky and not too dry: in case add flour or other milk as required.

Let's prepare the scones!

Go and spread the mixture on a floured surface and to a thickness of at least 2 centimeters. With the help of a pasta bowl (with a diameter of about 4 cm) cut some shapes that you will then put on a baking sheet covered with baking paper. Bake at 175 ° C, static oven, for about 20 minutes. At the end, let it cool and prepare a good tea.

23. VEGAN TEA COOKIES

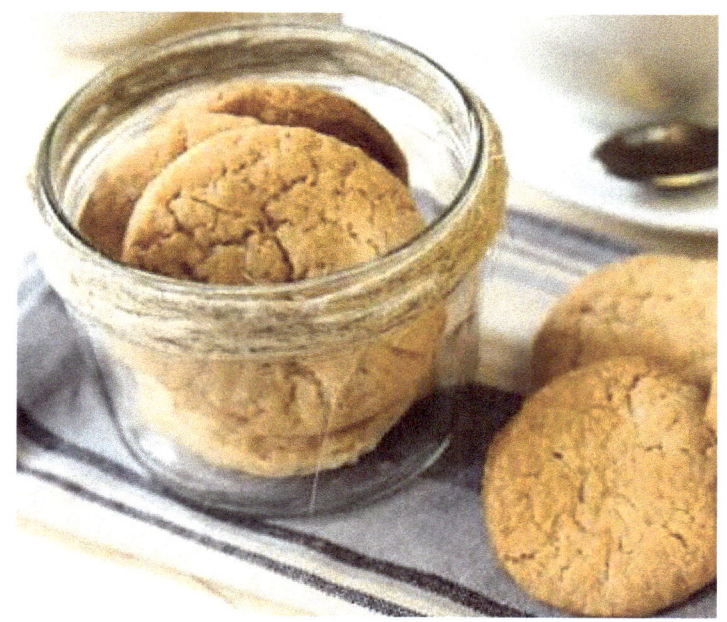

Ingredients

- 100 g of **wholemeal flour**
- 100 g of **rice flour**
- 70 ml **of sunflower** oil
- 50 ml **soy milk (or other vegetable milk)**
- 1 teaspoon of baking powder or **cream of tartar**
- 4 or g of whole cane sugar
- 1 tablespoon of **barley malt**

PREPARATION!

Flours

First, in a large bowl, sift the rice flour with the yeast and add the wholemeal one (do not sift the latter to avoid retaining some important elements during the operation). Add the brown sugar (you can also decide to chop it with a food processor, but it depends on the consistency of the biscuit you want to obtain, more or less rustic).

Off with the malt

Now add barley malt to the powders (you can also use rice malt, or, for a vegetarian version, wildflower honey), oil and milk. Start mixing everything well, taking care to mix all the ingredients perfectly. Then let the dough rest for about 15/20 minutes wrapped in cling film in the refrigerator.

Do we make cookies?

Now that the dough is ready, start rolling it out with the help of a rolling pin on a lightly floured pastry board and start making the biscuits with a round pastry cutter. Obviously you can decide to make the shape you prefer but remember that the more "complex" the shape, the more the cooking times will change, which you will have to personally verify. In the case of round biscuits of about 5 cm in diameter, proceed and place them on a dripping pan covered with parchment paper and bake them for 10/12 minutes at 180 ° C in a static oven. You just have to boil the water for tea.

24. VEGAN LASAGNA WITH SHIITAKE MUSHROOMS

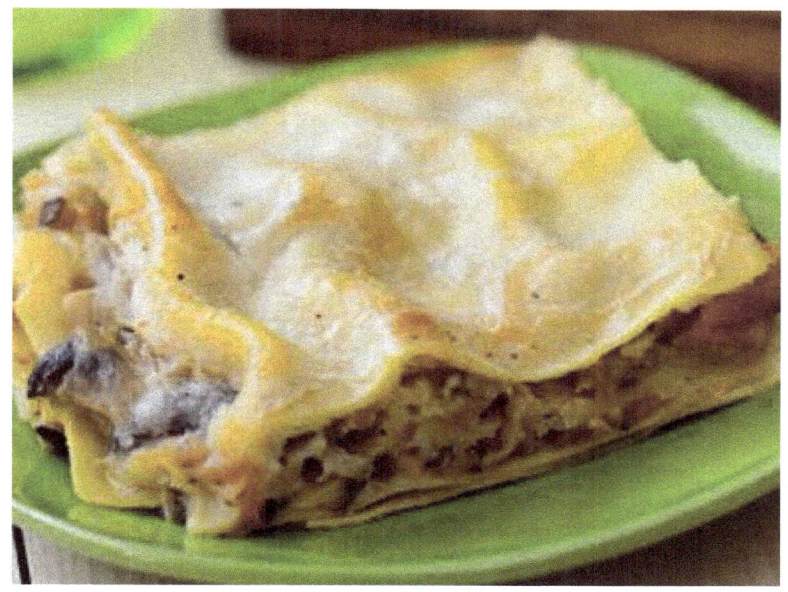

Ingredients

250 g fresh pasta without eggs
50 g of white flour
500 ml of **soy milk** unsweetened
50 g of extra virgin olive oil
1 onion
40 g mushroom **shiitake**
350 g of **carrots**
350 g of **zucchini**
400 g of **tomatoes**
nutmeg
salt and **pepper**
extra virgin olive oil

Tools

Pyrex dish

PREPARATION!

We prepare the mushrooms

Wash and let the mushrooms soak for about 1 hour. Chop them into cubes together with the vegetables that you have carefully washed. Brown the onion in a drizzle of hot oil and add all the vegetables at the end. Cook until soft and, if necessary, add a little water. At this point, add salt and pepper.

Off with the bechamel!

Prepare the béchamel by putting the flour, soy milk, oil in a saucepan and bringing everything almost to a boil (about 90 degrees), taking care to continue stirring to ensure that the ingredients all mix evenly. Remember that if you want a thicker béchamel you have to add flour, if you want it, however, more liquid, add milk.

And now let's do the layers

Place the fresh pasta on the bottom of the pan that you have greased with a drizzle of oil. Cover with a layer of vegetables and a layer of bechamel. Continue like this until all the vegetables and béchamel are completely gone. Bake the lasagna in a preheated oven at 180 degrees for 30 minutes.

25. VEGAN BANANA AND MATCHA TEA PLUMCAKE

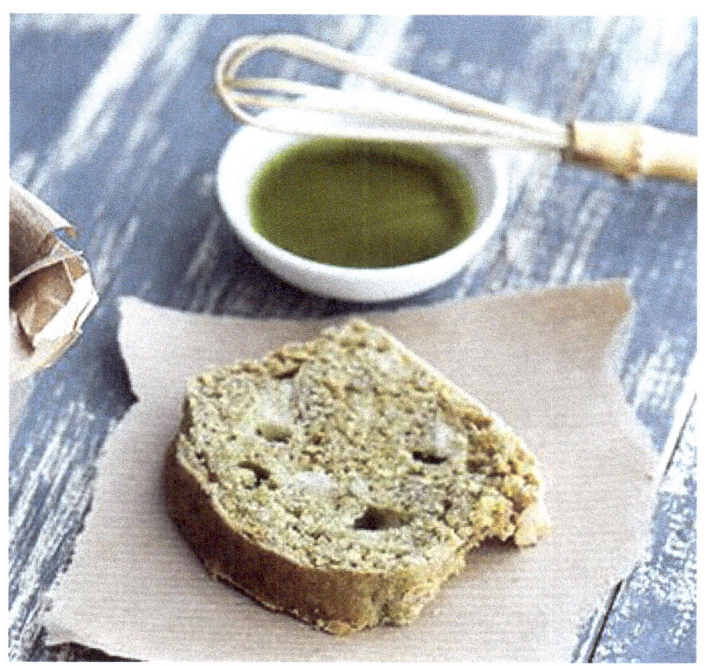

Ingredients

- 210 g flour
- 80 g semi wholemeal flour
- 1 large teaspoon of Matcha tea
- 1 sachet of **cream** of **tartar**
- 2 ripe bananas
- 1 pinch of salt
- 120 g of **maple syrup**
- 120 g of **rice milk**

- 40 g   of corn oil

PREPARATION!

We prepare the dough

First sift the flour, yeast and tea in a large bowl. Add a pinch of salt and then mix the powders together.
Separately, mix the liquid ingredients together and mash the bananas with a fork: combine all the ingredients, stirring quickly and vigorously so as to mix everything well.

We put in the mold and bake

Carefully pour the mixture into a loaf pan that you have oiled and floured first. Then bake at 180 ° C in a static oven for about 40 minutes. To check the cooking always use the good old toothpick test.

26. SEITAN ESCALOPES WITH GRAPES

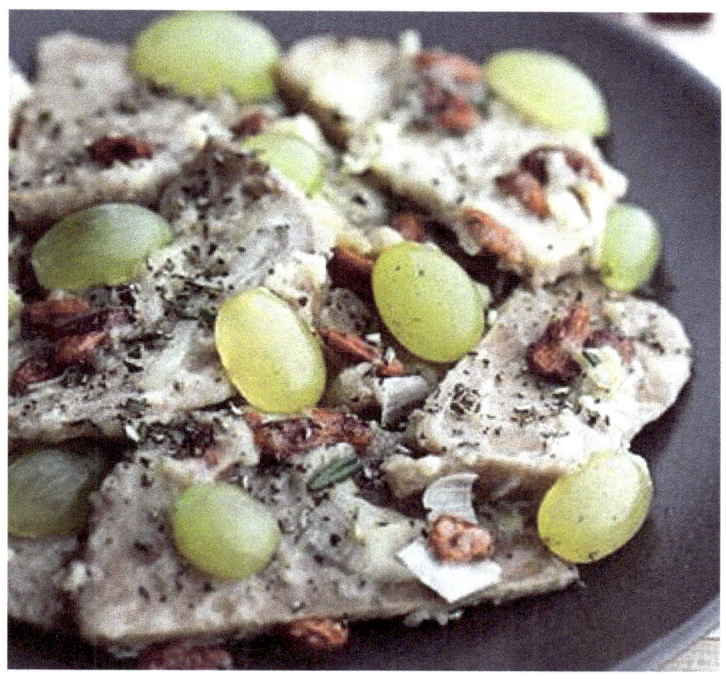

Ingredients

- 240 g natural **seitan** (1 pack)
- 20 g of **goji berries**
- 20 acini d ' **grape** white or 100 g of d' juice **grape**
- 1/2 **leek**
- fresh **rosemary**
- Provencal herbs to taste
- **rice flour to** taste
- extra virgin olive oil
- salt and **pepper**

PREPARATION!

The grape

Finely chop the fresh rosemary and add it to a spoonful of Provencal herbs. In a large container, mix the herbs with the rice flour. Set aside some chopped rosemary for the final garnish. Separately, with a centrifuge or a potato masher, extract their juice from the grapes. If you don't have fresh fruit, you can obviously use the juice that you commonly find in organic shops.

The seitan

Cut the seitan into slices about 5 mm thick and pass them in the mix of flour and spices in order to bread each individual slice very well. Press gently so that the flour adheres very well to the seitan. In a pan, heat a drizzle of oil and sauté the sliced leek and the goji berries. As soon as the leek has taken a little color, add the slices of seitan and shortly after the grape juice. Continue to cook over medium heat for about 10 minutes, adding a little hot water if the juice gets too dry. Season with salt and pepper and serve with chopped rosemary.

27. **VEGAN GRATED CHEESE**

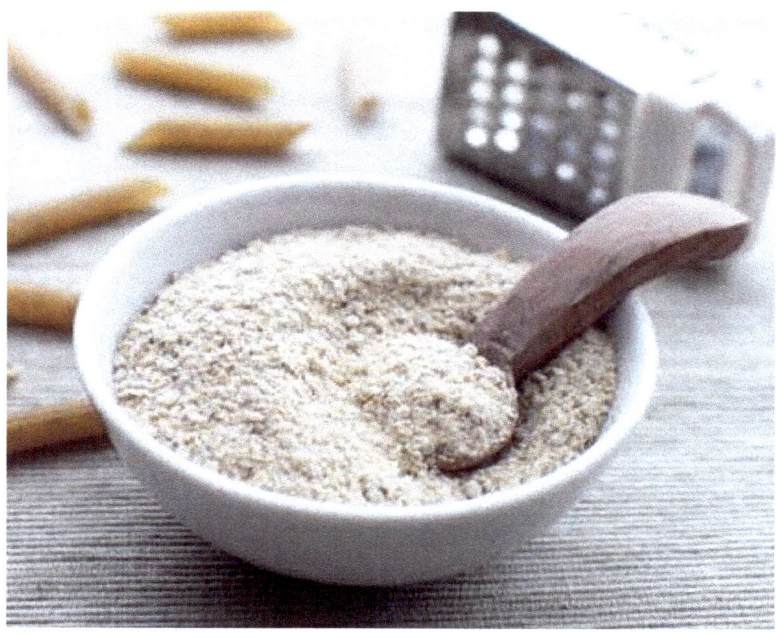

Ingredients

- 20 g of **nutritional yeast flakes**
- 30 g of **wheat germ**
- 20 g of **sesame seeds**
- 10 g of fine salt

PREPARATION!

The preparation is really simple: pour all the ingredients into the food processor and blend them until you get a fairly fine grain. It is advisable to use a powerful food processor to be able to pulverize the sesame seeds. To make sure that they release their full flavor, first toast the sesame seeds in a non-stick pan: they will be ready when they start to turn slightly golden.

28. VEGAN PUDDING WITH PEARS AND GOJI BERRIES

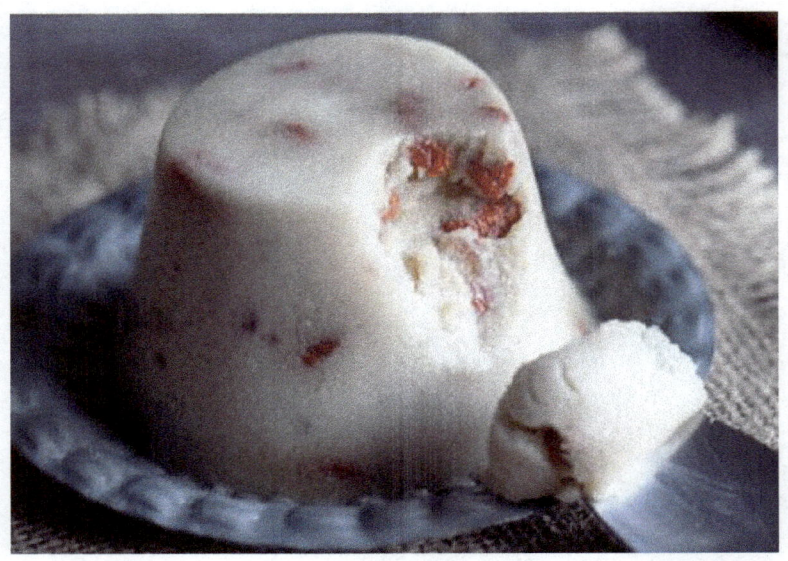

Ingredients

- 100 g of **rice flour**
- 500 g of **rice milk**
- 70 g of brown sugar
- 50 g of **Goji berries**
- 1 pear (about 50 g of pulp)
- 30 g of candied fruit
- 1/2 teaspoon of **agar agar**

PREPARATION!

Berries and milk

Soak the Goji berries in warm water for about 10 minutes. In a saucepan pour the milk and bring to a boil; add the rice flour and agar agar (which you have previously diluted in a drop of milk) continuing to mix with a whisk to avoid the formation of lumps.

The cooking

Now, continue adding the sugar and cook until the cream begins to thicken, then turn off the heat and add the drained Goji berries, the candied fruit and the diced pear. At this point you just have to mix the ingredients, then pour the mixture into 4 aluminum muffin molds and let it cool in the refrigerator until firm (about 2 hours)

29. VEGAN SPREADABLE CHEESE

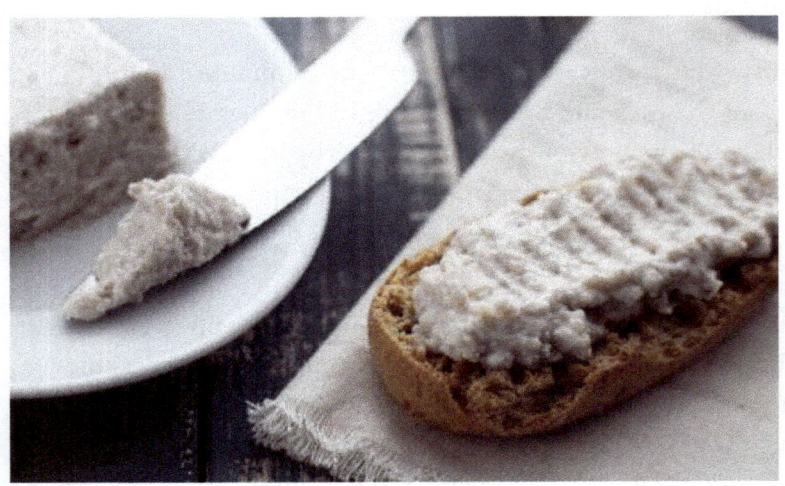

Ingredients

- 30 g of 5 cereal flakes
- 400 g of **soy milk**
- 40 g of **nutritional yeast**
- 30 g of **tahini** (**sesame** cream)
- 20 g of **corn starch** (or cornstarch)
- 8 g of **agar agar** (about 2 teaspoons)
- 1 tablespoon of lemon **juice**
- 1 pinch of salt
- extra virgin olive oil

PREPARATION!

We blend the ingredients

Make the cereal flakes flour in a food processor and then, slowly, while running the robot at low speed, combine the other ingredients: about 3/4 of the soy milk, yeast, tahini, starch, lemon and finally the salt.

We add the agar agar

Dissolve the agar agar in the remaining soy milk and add it to the other ingredients. Put the mixture thus obtained in a saucepan and let it thicken over low heat.

Let it cool down

Pour the mixture into a previously oiled mold or into individual muffin molds. Leave to cool covered to room temperature and then at least 2 hours in the refrigerator.

30. RISOTTO WITH BLUEBERRIES AND PORCINI MUSHROOMS

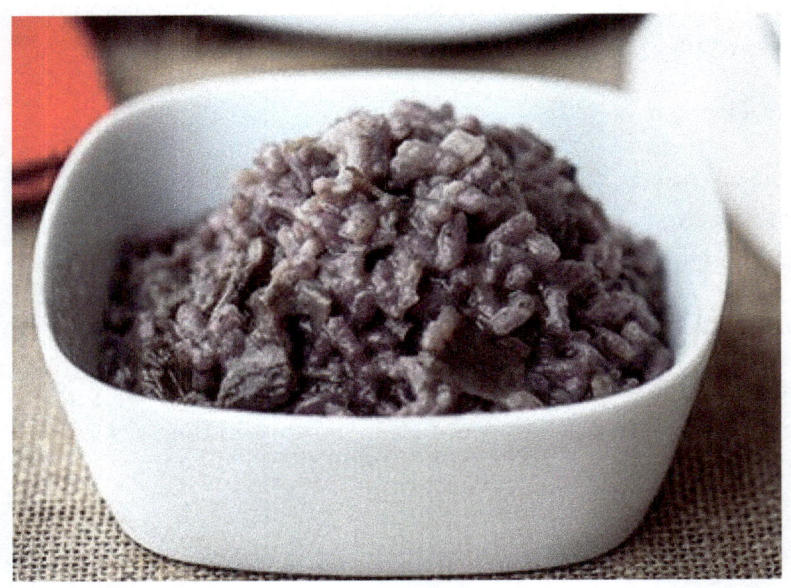

Ingredients

- 320 g of Vialone rice
- extra virgin olive oil
- 1/2 chopped onion
- 1/2 glass of dry white wine
- 50 g of blueberries
- 40 gr of dried porcini mushrooms
- **vegetable broth to** taste
- salt

PREPARATION!

Step 1 - The preparations

In a bowl, soak the mushrooms with warm water for about 15 minutes. Meanwhile, prepare the vegetable broth.

Step **2 - Let's roll up our sleeves**

In a saucepan, brown the chopped onion in oil; as soon as it takes a little color, pour in the rice and toast it for a couple of minutes. Add the wine and wait for it to evaporate completely. Cover the rice with the vegetable broth and start mixing. Add the mushrooms, after having drained them, and continue to cook for about 18 minutes, adding the broth as often as needed.

Step 3 - Final touch

- About 5 minutes before the end of cooking, add the blueberries and finish cooking. Turn off the heat.
  Dissolve some salt in a little broth and pour it over the rice while continuing to mix. Finally, stir in the extra virgin olive oil or if you want to give a frothier consistency with vegetable butter or **soy cream**.

31. SPINACH AND TOFU ROLLS

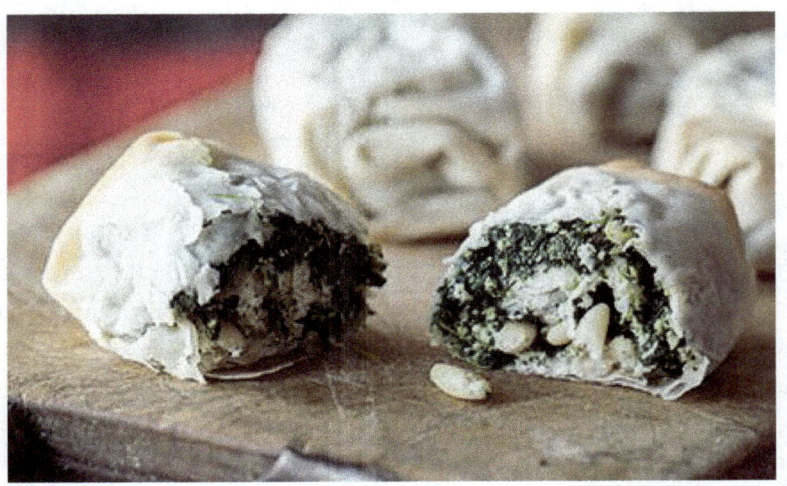

Ingredients

- 16 sheets of phyllo dough (15 × 24 cm)
- 500 g of fresh spinach
- 25 g of **pine nuts**
- 125 g of **tofu**
- the zest of 1 **lemon**
- **nutmeg to** taste
- **fresh ginger to** taste
- extra virgin olive oil to taste
- salt and **pepper**

PREPARATION!

We boil the spinach

- Carefully wash the spinach and cook them in plenty of salted water. Let them cool and squeeze them thoroughly to remove excess water.

Let's skip the tofu

- Meanwhile, sauté the crumbled tofu in a non-stick pan (you can do it with your hands) together with a drizzle of extra virgin olive oil. Add the spinach, black pepper, grated ginger, lemon zest and nutmeg. Mix thoroughly and season with salt. Aside, toast the pine nuts that you add to the other ingredients quickly and without other fats.

We prepare the rolls

- Cut out rectangles measuring 15 × 24 cm from the sheets of phyllo dough and overlap them in pairs on a cutting board or on a smooth surface. Remember to cover the remaining sheets of phyllo dough while cutting the others because this dough is very delicate and tends to dry out very easily (you can cover it with some film or a slightly damp clean cloth). Distribute 2 tablespoons of dough in the center, fold the four edges inwards for about 1 cm and then roll them up into rolls.

In the oven!

- Brush the surface with extra virgin olive oil and bake at 200 degrees for about 10 minutes, static oven, taking care not to burn the ends of the phyllo dough.

32. VEGAN ALSATIAN APPLE PIE

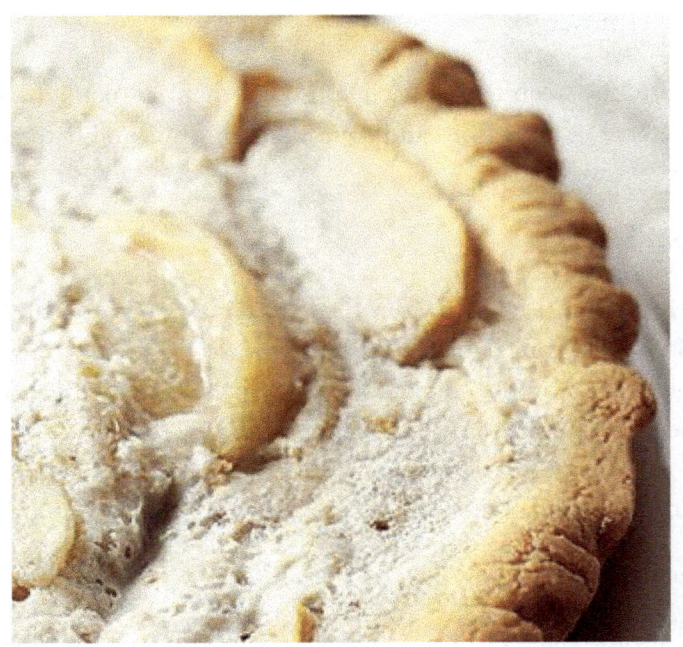

Ingredients

For the pastry

- 200 g of flour type 0
- 50 g of **wholemeal spelled flour**
- 60 g of **malt**
- 60 ml of corn oil
- 70 ml of warm water
- 1 pinch of salt
- 1 teaspoon of **cream** of **tartar**

For the stuffing

- 500 g of Fuji **apples** (about 2 **apples**)
- sugar-free **apricot** jam
- 50 g of brown sugar
- 100 ml of **vegetable cream**
- 20 g of **rice flour**
- 1 **Tonka bean**
- **soy milk to** taste

PREPARATION!

Let's prepare the pastry

- In a large bowl, combine all the dry ingredients then sift the flours to make the mixture free of lumps. Separately, mix the oil with the malt and water which you will then add to the other ingredients.
  Mix everything well and knead the dough for a few minutes. At the end you will have to have a homogeneous and elastic dough that you will have to rest in the refrigerator, covered, for at least 1 hour.

Shortcrust pastry cooking

- Roll out the pastry in a tart tin, peel the apples and cut them into thin slices. Spread the jam on the bottom of the pastry and cover with the apple slices. Bake at 180 ° C for about 15 minutes.

Last step

- Now prepare a fairly liquid cream with the other ingredients: mix the cream with the rice flour and sugar. Grate the Tonka bean and mix the ingredients by adding a lot of milk when needed to dilute the cream. If you don't have beans, you can replace them with a little vanilla pod (dissolve the seeds in the liquid mixture). Pour the freshly prepared cream over the cake and put it back in the oven for another 15 minutes. At the end of cooking, let it cool and serve.

33. **LIME FLAVORED MUSHROOM CROUTONS**

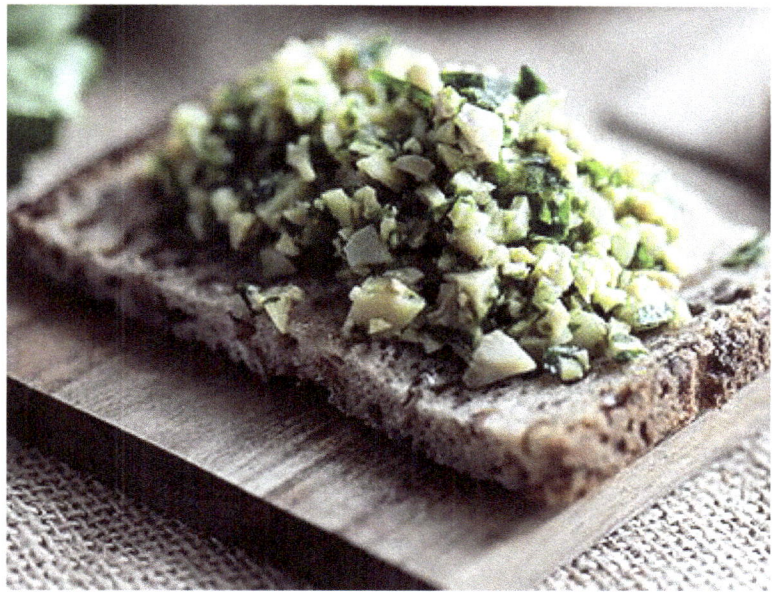

Ingredients

- sliced rye bread
- 20 champignon mushrooms in oil
- 1 bunch of parsley
- **chives to** taste
- 1 **lime** (zest and juice)
- salt and **pepper**

PREPARATION!

Let's prepare the ingredients

- Drain very well and chop the champignon mushrooms. Clean and finely chop the parsley and chives.

Mix all the ingredients, add the lime zest, a pinch of salt and pepper. If you don't have lime, you can use lemon.

We serve!

- From the rye bread, cut small rectangles into the shape and size you prefer, if you want you can also decide to toast them lightly. Divide the mushroom mixture on each of these and serve. You can also sprinkle some fresh parsley again at the top.

34. ORANGE MUFFINS AND TONKA BEANS

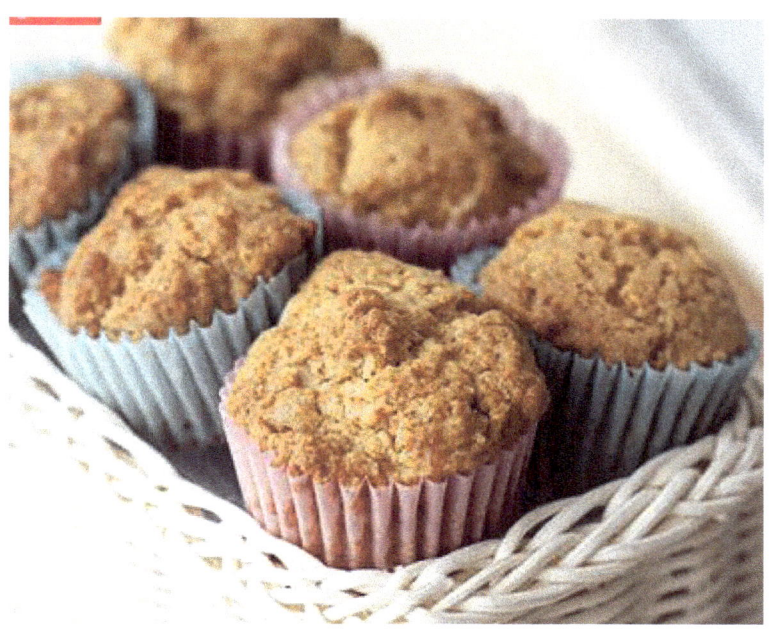

Ingredients

- 150 g of flour 00
- 150 g of whole meal **spelled flour**
- 1 pinch of salt
- 1 sachet of **cream** of **tartar**
- 1 **Tonka bean**
- zest of 1 **orange**
- 50 ml of orange **juice**
- 120 g of **agave syrup**
- 120 g of corn oil

PREPARATION!

Let's prepare the muffin dough

- In a large bowl, mix the dry ingredients of the recipe together: then add the sifted flour, a pinch of salt, cream of tartar, zest and grated Tonka bean. In another bowl, add the liquid ingredients, then the oil, orange juice and agave syrup.

Let's mix and bake!

- Let's combine all the ingredients: take the liquids, add them to the powders and start mixing. Once you have a homogeneous mixture, pour it into muffin cups of the size you prefer, taking care to fill them up to halfway. Bake in a static oven at 180 degrees for 25 minutes

35. VEGAN LASAGNA WITH ESCAROLE, OLIVES AND WALNUTS

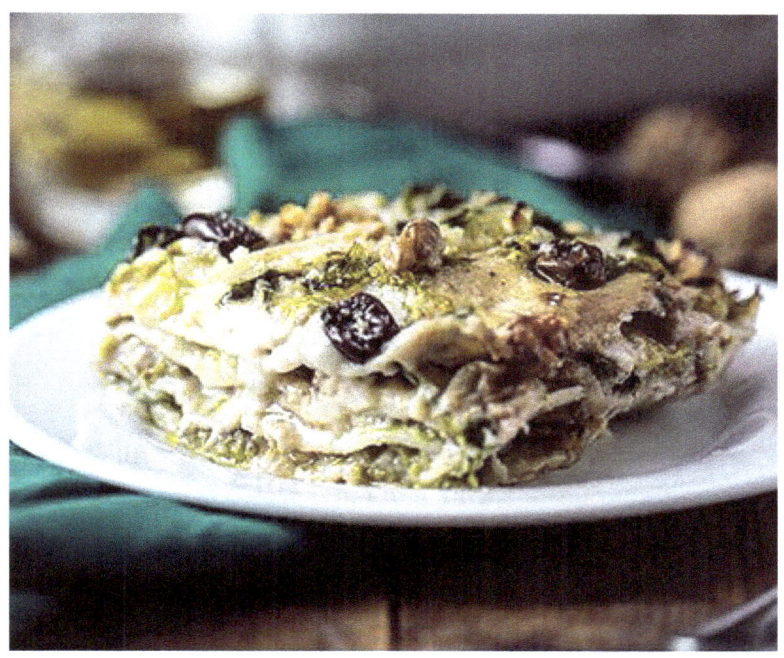

Ingredients

- 250 g of lasagna without eggs
- 1 kg of escarole
- 1 onion
- 1 clove of garlic
- 750 g of soy milk not sweetened
- 50 g of flour 0
- 50 g of olive oil
- 1 tablespoon of nutritional yeast
- 60 g of walnuts
- 80 g of Taggiasca olives
- Vegetable grated cheese
- nutmeg

- Salt and pepper

PREPARATION!

- Start by chopping the onion and frying it in a large non-stick pan or wok along with the garlic clove. Cut the escarole into strips and wash it well, then drain it as much as possible from the water. Add the salad to the pan and sauté over medium-high heat until it is wilted and a little water has dried.

We bake

- Bake your lasagna in a preheated static oven at 200 ° C for 30 minutes, then take it out of the oven and let it cool for a couple of minutes before serving cut into slices.

36. **VEGAN LASAGNA WITH BROCCOLI, WALNUTS AND SUNFLOWER SEEDS**

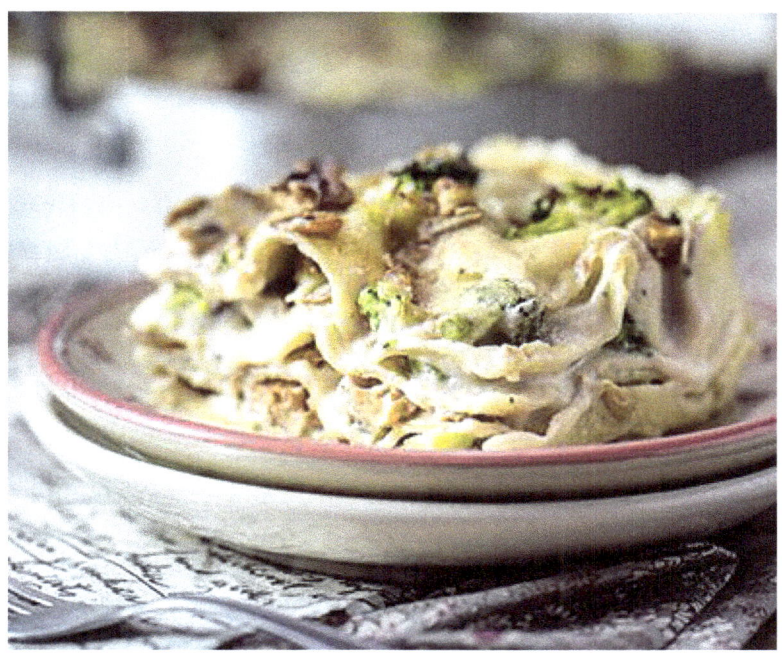

Ingredients

- 250 g of semolina lasagna
- 1 large broccoli
- 50 g of walnuts
- 40 g of sunflower seeds
- 1 pinch of paprika
- ½ teaspoon of chopped rosemary

for the bechamel:

- 750 g of soy milk not sweetened
- 60 g of flour 0

- 30 g of extra virgin olive oil
- 30 g of sunflower oil
- 1 tablespoon of nutritional yeast
- nutmeg
- Salt and pepper

PREPARATION!

- Start by washing the broccoli well, divide it into fairly small florets and blanch them in lightly salted boiling water for a few minutes, just long enough to soften them, then drain and let them cool on a plate.

We toast the sunflower seeds

- Toast the sunflower seeds in a very hot non-stick pan with a drop of oil, the paprika, the rosemary and a pinch of salt until golden brown.

We boil the pasta

- Boil the lasagna 3-4 at a time for 3 minutes in the water in which you cooked the broccoli, adding a tablespoon of seed oil so that they do not stick and gradually transferring them to a work surface covered with parchment paper.

Let's prepare the bechamel

- Now take care of the béchamel: heat the two types of oil and the flour in a saucepan and let it fry for a couple of minutes. Then pour in the hot soy milk, stirring constantly with a wooden spoon or a whisk in order to incorporate the soy milk with roux well without leaving lumps. Once all the milk has been combined, season with salt, pepper, nutmeg and nutritional yeast and bring to a boil.

Let's assemble the lasagna

- At this point all that remains is to assemble your lasagna. Pour a couple of spoonfuls of béchamel into the bottom of a baking dish, arrange a layer of lasagna, cover with the béchamel and stuff with broccoli, toasted sunflower seeds and coarsely chopped walnuts. Continue with the succession of layers until all the ingredients are used up, then pour half a cup of water into the corners of the pan.

We bake

- Bake your lasagna in a preheated static oven at 180 ° C for 30 minutes and take it out of the oven once the dough is soft and the surface slightly golden, let it rest for a minute and serve hot.

37. CREAM OF CARROTS AND PEANUT BUTTER WITH SPICED CROUTONS

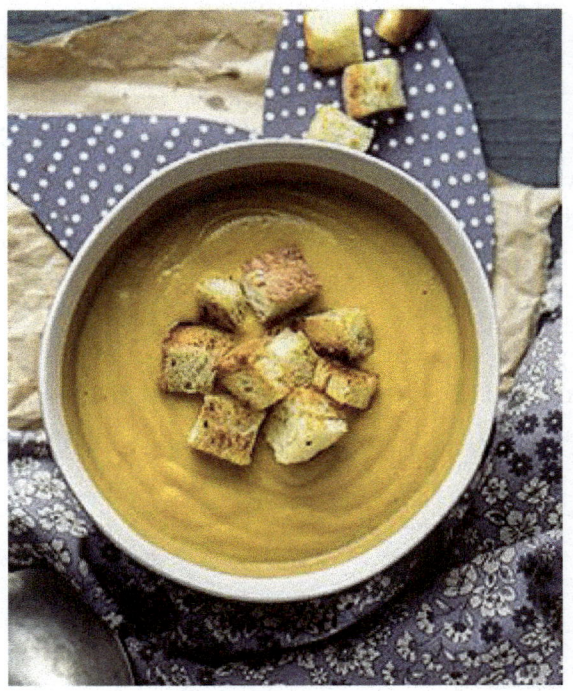

Ingredients

- 500 g of carrots
- 1 onion
- 2 potatoes
- 1 teaspoon of chopped rosemary
- 60 g of peanut butter
- vegetable broth
- salt and pepper
- 2 slices of bread
- 1 clove of garlic
- 1 pinch of red pepper

PREPARATION!

- Start by cleaning the onion and reducing it into cubes, then heat a large pot, pour a drizzle of oil and fry the onion. Meanwhile, peel and cut the potatoes into cubes and add them to the pot together with the onions, add salt and cook for 5 minutes.

PREPARATION the vegetables

- Peel and chop the carrots as well and add them to the rest of the vegetables along with the rosemary. Leave to flavor for a couple of minutes then cover everything with vegetable broth and let it boil for about 20 minutes, or until the vegetables are cooked.

Let's add the peanut butter

- Turn off the heat, then add the peanut butter and blend everything with the hand blender until you get a perfectly smooth cream.

We prepare the croutons

- For the croutons, cut the bread into not too large cubes, heat a non-stick pan with a drizzle of oil, a clove of garlic and a pinch of chilli and once the oil is hot, add the bread. Fry for a few minutes, turning the croutons often, so that they brown evenly on all sides.

38. VEGAN LASAGNA WITH PUMPKIN AND TURNIP GREENS WITH OATMEAL BECHAMEL

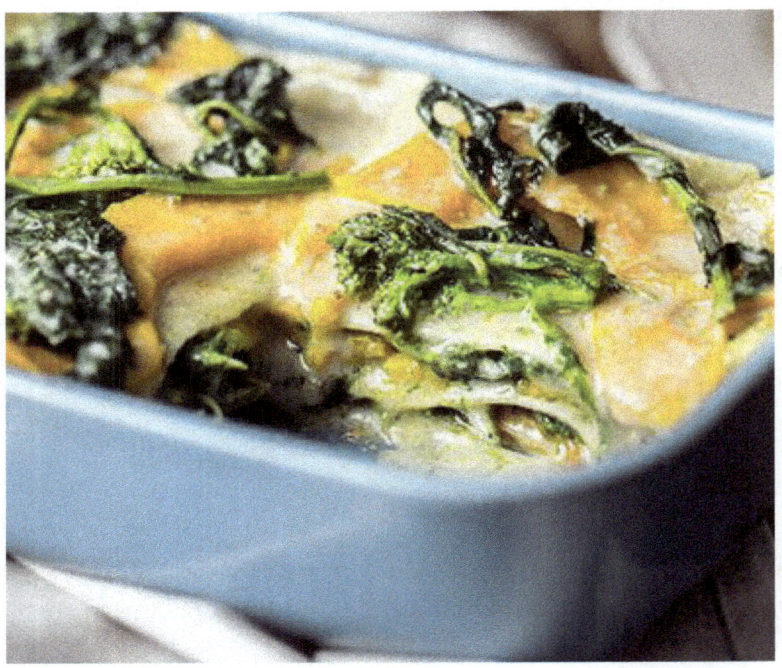

Ingredients

- 300 g of egg-free lasagna sheet
- 500 g of turnip greens
- 400 g of pumpkin
- 1 clove of garlic
- 1 sprig of rosemary
- A pinch of cinnamon
- for the oat sauce
- 500 ml oat milk unsweetened
- 40 g of flour 2
- 20 g of extra virgin olive oil

- 20 g of sunflower oil
- 1 tablespoon of nutritional yeast
- nutmeg
- Salt and pepper

PREPARATION!

First the béchamel

- In a saucepan pour the flour 2 and the two types of oil, mix well with a wooden spoon and put on medium heat. As soon as the roux starts to sizzle, add the hot oat milk slowly, continuing to stir constantly to avoid the formation of lumps. Always continuing to mix, bring the béchamel to a boil and cook for at least 2 minutes. Turn off the heat and season with salt, pepper, nutmeg and nutritional yeast.

We roast the pumpkin

- Clean the pumpkin from internal filaments and seeds, remove the peel and cut it into 2-3 mm thin slices. Arrange them on a baking sheet lined with parchment paper, season with salt, oil, a sprinkle of cinnamon and finely chopped rosemary. Bake in a static oven at 200 ° C for 10 minutes.

Let's cook the turnip greens

- Clean and wash the turnip greens, cut them in half and blanch them in lightly salted boiling water for a couple of minutes. Drain them well, then sauté them in a pan with a drizzle of oil in which you have sautéed a clove of garlic. Season with salt, pepper and nutmeg and turn off the heat.

Let's assemble the lasagna

- Boil the lasagna sheets in abundant salted water for 3 minutes, then drain and arrange them on a tray. Cover the bottom of a pan with a few tablespoons of bechamel, arrange a layer of pasta, cover with bechamel and then a layer of pumpkin and turnip greens. Proceed with another layer of pasta and repeat the previous layers until all the ingredients are used up. Finish with a layer of vegetables lightly covered with béchamel in order to keep them visible but soft.

And now in the oven

- Bake the lasagna in a static oven at 180 ° C for 20 minutes. Once ready, take them out of the oven, let them cool for 10 minutes and serve.

39. POLENTA VEGAN LASAGNA WITH RADICCHIO AND MUSHROOMS

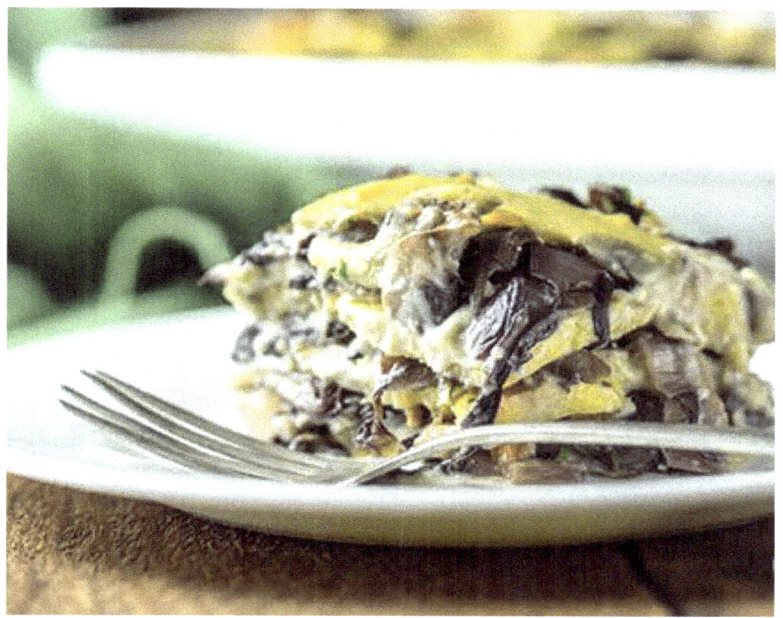

Ingredients

- 200 g of polenta flour
- 800 g of water
- 3 tablespoons of extra virgin olive oil
- 1 pinch of salt
- for the bechamel:
- 500 g of soy milk not sweetened
- 25 g of corn starch
- 20 g of extra virgin olive oil
- 20 g of sunflower oil
- 2 tablespoons of nutritional yeast
- nutmeg

- Salt and pepper
- for the dressing:
- 400 g of mushrooms
- 1 - 2 heads of long radicchio
- 1 teaspoon of chopped rosemary
- 1 tablespoon of chopped parsley
- 2 cloves of garlic
- 50 g of hazelnuts

PREPARATION!

- Start by preparing the polenta: bring the water to a boil, then add salt and add the oil and the corn flour, keeping everything mixed with a whisk to avoid the formation of lumps. Dip a wooden spoon under water and use it to stir the polenta from time to time, and cook for 45 minutes.

We prepare the vegetables

- Clean the mushrooms with a damp cloth and remove the ends of the stems. Slice them and sauté them in a pan with a drizzle of oil and a clove of garlic, keeping the heat high so that they brown. Once cooked, turn off the heat and season with salt, pepper and parsley. Separately, slice the radicchio into strips at least 1 cm thick, wash it and dry it well with a centrifuge. Then sauté it in a pan over high heat with a drizzle of oil, a clove of garlic and the chopped rosemary until wilted.

Now the bechamel

- Dissolve the starch in a small bowl with a drop of soy milk, then pour the rest of the milk into a saucepan together with the two types of oil and bring to a boil. Now add the dissolved starch, mixing well and cook for a few more minutes until the béchamel has thickened slightly. Season with nutritional yeast, salt, pepper and nutmeg to taste and set aside.

Let's assemble the lasagna

- Cut the cold polenta into thin slices then compose your lasagna by pouring a spoonful of bechamel on the bottom of your pan, arrange a layer of slices of polenta and cover with bechamel, mushrooms, radicchio and chopped hazelnuts. Repeat the succession of layers until all ingredients are used up, finishing with a thin layer of béchamel on the last layer to keep your lasagna soft. Bake in a static oven at 200 ° C for 15 minutes, take them out of the oven and let them cool for a few minutes before serving them cut into slices.

40. ORECCHIETTE WITH PEPPER CREAM

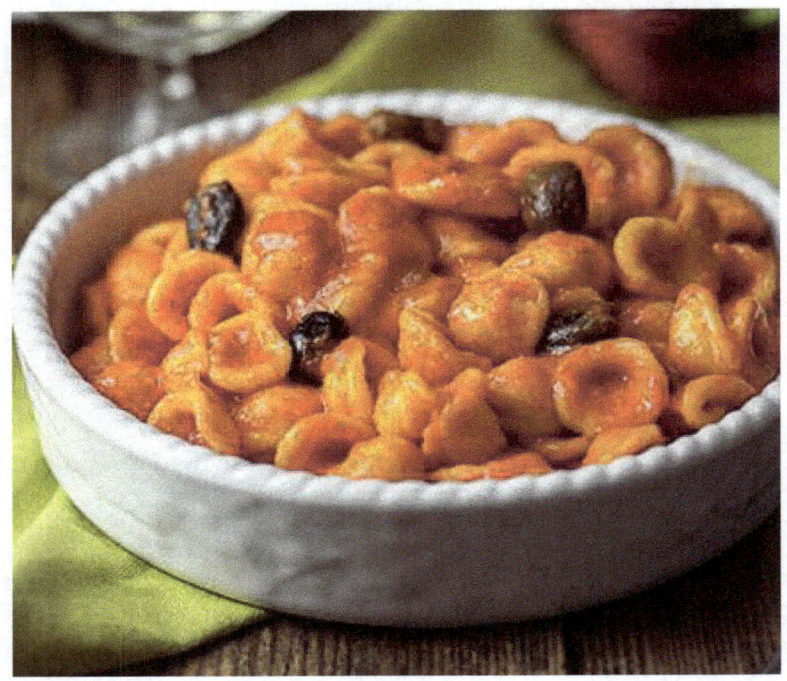

Ingredients

- 500 g of fresh orecchiette
- 2 red peppers
- 1 clove of garlic
- 1 teaspoon of miso (rice or barley)
- 80 g of Taggiasca olives
- 100 ml of soy cream
- ½ teaspoon of paprika

PREPARATION!

- Wash the peppers well, remove the stalk, seeds and internal white filaments then cut them into cubes. In a non-stick pan, fry the garlic clove with a drop of oil and once golden add the peppers. Season with a pinch of salt and paprika and cook for about 15 minutes until soft, adding a drop of water if necessary to prevent them from burning.

We whisk the pepper cream

- Boil the orecchiette in plenty of lightly salted water and drain when al dente. Meanwhile, transfer the peppers to the blender along with the soy cream and miso and blend until perfectly smooth.

We season the pasta

- Put the cream back into the pan, add the olives and let it cook over medium heat for a couple of minutes. At this point add the orecchiette and sauté for another couple of minutes, until the sauce is a little narrow and has formed a nice soft cream. Serve your orecchiette hot immediately.

41. **VEGAN TART WITH TURMERIC CREAM**

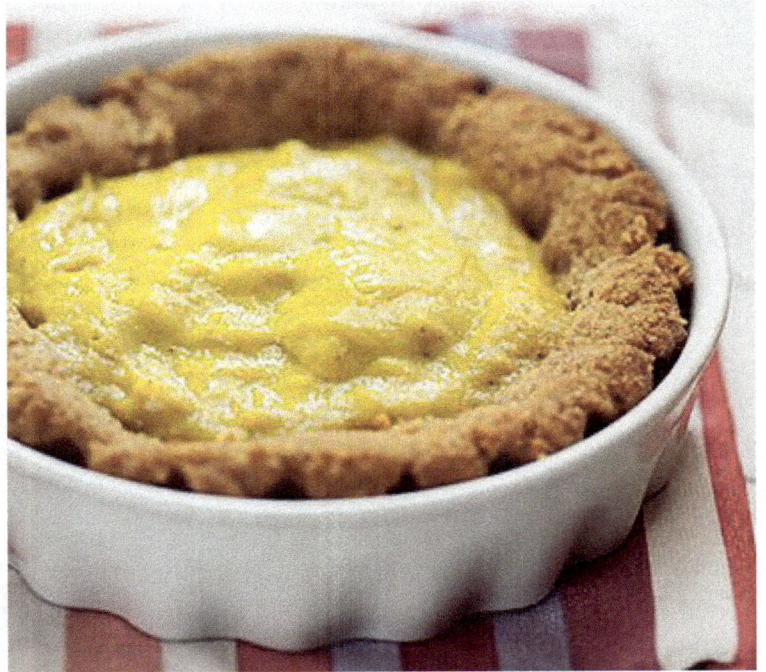

Ingredients

For the pastry

- 150 g of wholemeal spelled flour
- 100 g of corn meal 's foil
- 60 g of rice malt
- 50 g of corn oil
- 50 g of lukewarm water
- 1 pinch of salt
- 1/2 sachet of cream of tartar

For the cream

- 500 g of spelled milk

- 100 g vegetable cream
- 40 g of brown rice flour
- 100 g of refined cane sugar
- 4 g of turmeric

PREPARATION!

- Let's prepare the pastry
- Combine all the dry ingredients in a bowl. Separately, mix the oil with the malt and then add them together with the water in the bowl with the other ingredients. Mix everything well and knead the dough for a few minutes.
- At the end you will have to have a crumbly dough that you will have to rest for an hour in the refrigerator.

We prepare the cream

- In a saucepan, add the milk, sugar and turmeric. Melt the sugar when cold then turn on the heat and at a moderate flame add the rice flour and vegetable cream.
- Bring to a boil, taking care to stir constantly to prevent the cream from burning on the bottom of the saucepan. Lower the heat slightly and continue until the cream thickens.

PREPARATION OF the pastry

- Take the dough from the refrigerator and roll it out in a tart pan. Prick the bottom and cover it with dried beans or rice. This will help keep the dough from growing excessively.
- Bake in a static oven at 180 ° C for 20 minutes and then let it cool down.

42. **ZUCCHINI WITH MANGO AND APPLES**

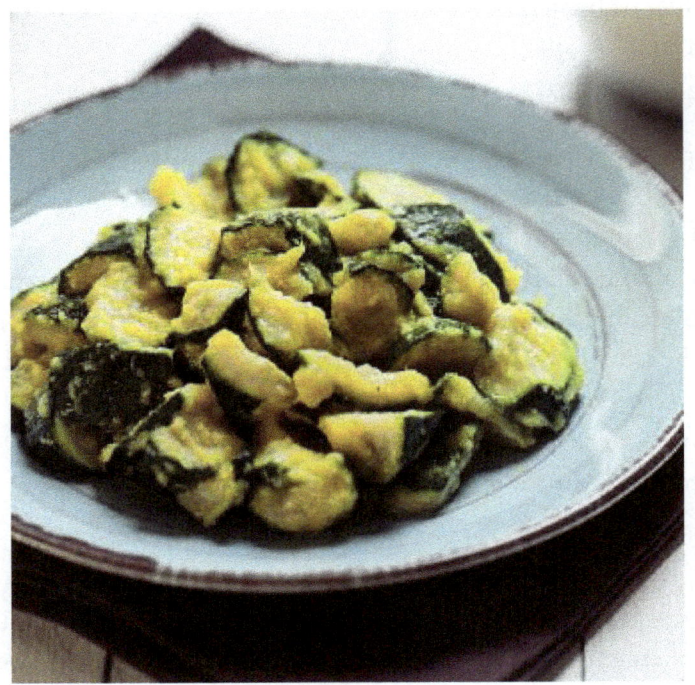

Ingredients

- 2 fuji apples
- 1 mango
- 4 courgettes
- hot water to taste
- extra virgin olive oil
- green curry

PREPARATION!

We prepare fruit and vegetables

- Peel the apples and mango and cut them into coarse cubes. In a non-stick pan, heat a drizzle of extra virgin olive oil and add the cut fruit. Blanch it for a few minutes, then pour a drizzle of water to finish cooking: it must be soft but not pulped. A few minutes before the end of cooking, add the green curry diluted in a drop of hot water.

We sew vegetables

- With an immersion blender reduce everything to cream and if it is too thick we recommend adding a drop of apple juice. Now cut the courgettes coarsely and sauté a few minutes in a wok or, alternatively, in a non-stick pan with a drizzle of extra virgin olive oil. At the end of cooking they must still be crunchy; add salt if necessary. Finally, add the fruit cream to the zucchini, brown them for another minute in a pan and serve. You can also decide to serve the fruit cream separately and add it to the zucchini as you like.

43. QUINOA VEGAN BURGER

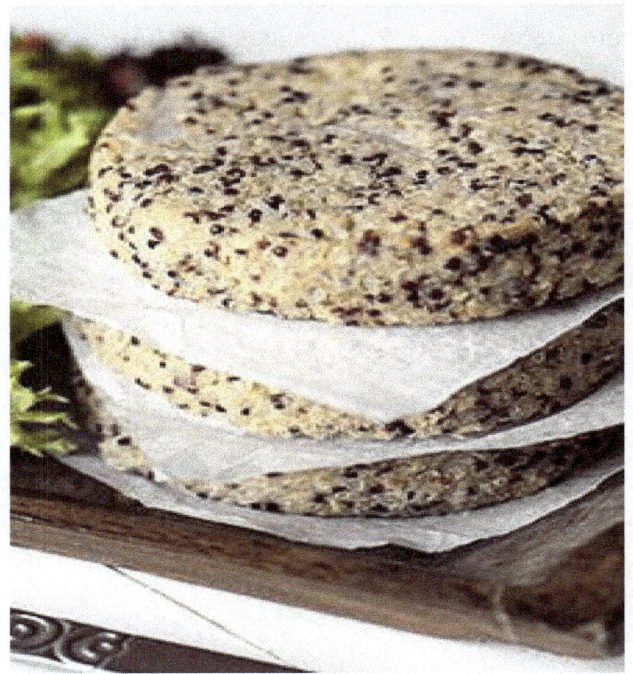

Ingredients

- 1 potato
- 200 g of quinoa
- 1 onion
- Provence herbs to taste
- chilli (optional)
- extra virgin olive oil to taste
- Salt to taste

PREPARATION!

- Cook the quinoa in 400 ml of cold water for about ten minutes. Over moderate heat, bring to a boil and continue to cook until the liquid is completely absorbed: let it cool. Separately, in more salted water, boil the potato and let it cool.

The other ingredients

- Separately, in a pan, brown the onion with a drizzle of extra virgin olive oil, add the spices and mix. Now pour all the ingredients into a bowl and mix them until you get a fairly homogeneous and workable mixture.

We form the burgers

- With wet hands or with the help of a circular pastry ring, shape burgers of the size you prefer and spread them out on a baking tray covered with baking paper. Bake at 200 ° C for about 10 minutes per side: they will have to take a little color on both sides.

44. **PUMPKIN, ROSEMARY, RAISINS AND CHOCOLATE MUFFINS**

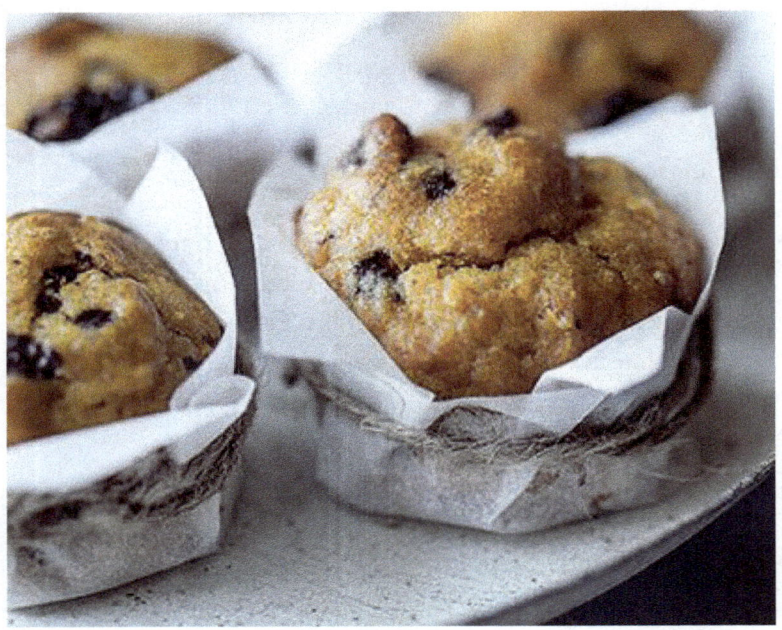

Ingredients

- 150 g of flour type 0
- a pinch of salt
- 1/2 sachet of natural yeast based on cream of tartar (8 g)
- 60 g of agave syrup
- 60 g of corn oil
- 250 g of boiled pumpkin
- 2 teaspoons of rosemary needles
- 50 g of dark chocolate
- 50 g of raisins

PREPARATION!

- First, sift the flour and sourdough into a large bowl to prevent lumps from forming. Separately, finely chop the dark chocolate and rosemary with a knife. Then, in a glass with warm water, soak the raisins for a few minutes to soften them and then squeeze them.
- Then blend the pumpkin, which you have previously boiled, and add the liquid ingredients. Mix them well and then pour them into the bowl together with the flour and baking powder.

We mix and ...

Then, mix vigorously and quickly. The time has come to add the chocolate, squeezed raisins and rosemary to your mixture: continue to mix trying to obtain a mixture as homogeneous as possible. Then pour it into a muffin mold and bake in a static oven at 180 ° C for about 30 minutes.

45. **PEAR AND CHOCOLATE VEGAN COOKIES**

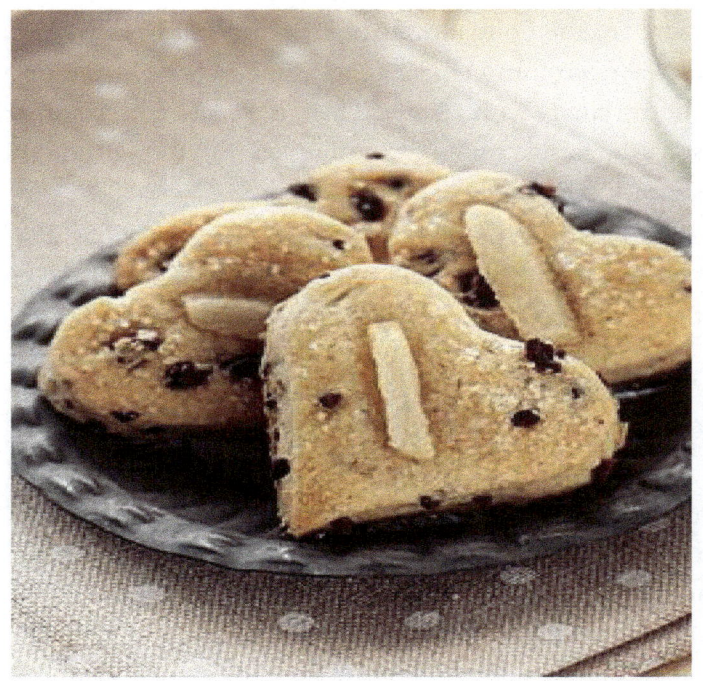

Ingredients

- 200 g of flour type 0
- 80 g of wholemeal flour
- 120 g of clear pear juice
- 1 teaspoon natural yeast based on cream of tartar
- 20 g of corn starch
- 1 pinch of salt
- 100 g of corn oil
- 50 g of whole cane sugar + sugar for decoration
- 40 g of cocoa bean grains
- 1/2 pear

PREPARATION!

The dough

- In a large bowl, sift the type 0 flour and baking powder. Add the whole meal flour, salt, sugar, cocoa, corn starch and mix well. Separately, add and mix the liquid ingredients: pear juice and corn oil. Knead the dough until a smooth and soft consistency is obtained, forming a loaf that must rest in the refrigerator for at least 30 minutes.

The cooking

- At the end of the rest period, take the dough, roll it out on a surface covered with baking paper and cut out some biscuits with pastry rings of different shapes. Now place the biscuits on a baking tray covered with baking paper and on each place some slices of fresh pear cut into sticks. Sprinkle with brown sugar and bake at 180 ° C, static oven, for about 20/25 minutes. At the end, let it cool and serve.

46. WHOLEMEAL SHELLS WITH SAGE AND POTATOES

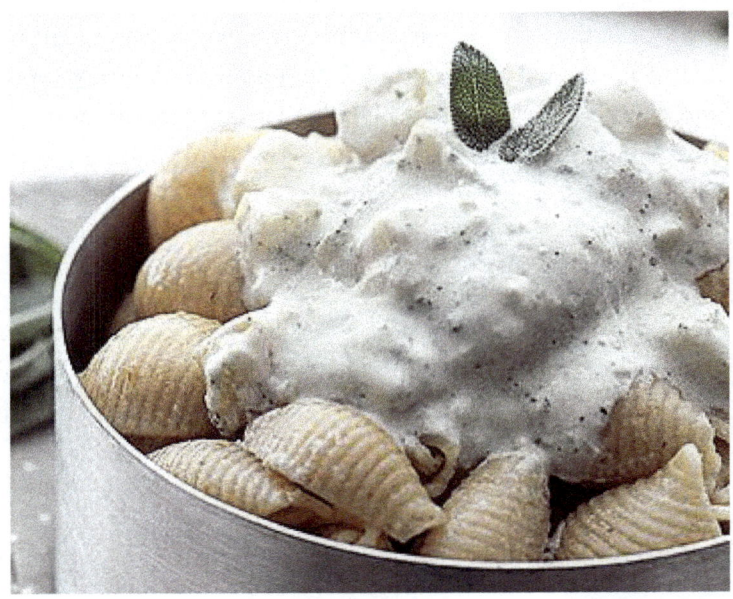

Ingredients

- 320 g of pasta like wholemeal shells
- 400 g of red potatoes
- 200 g of soy cream
- 6 sage leaves
- salt and pepper

PREPARATION!

Let's prepare the dressing

- Wash the potatoes under running water and cook them whole, with the peel, in plenty of salted water. Let them cool and cut them into cubes of about 1 centimeter. Wash the sage and sauté it in a non-stick pan with a drizzle of oil. Add the soy cream, mix and blend with an immersion robot. Add the potatoes and season with salt and pepper.

Pasta is... go!

- Cook the pasta in salted water, drain and season with the sage sauce and potatoes. You can choose the shape of pasta you prefer, we suggest a pasta that collects the sauce well like these wholemeal shells.

47. **MINT AND CHOCOLATE DONUTS**

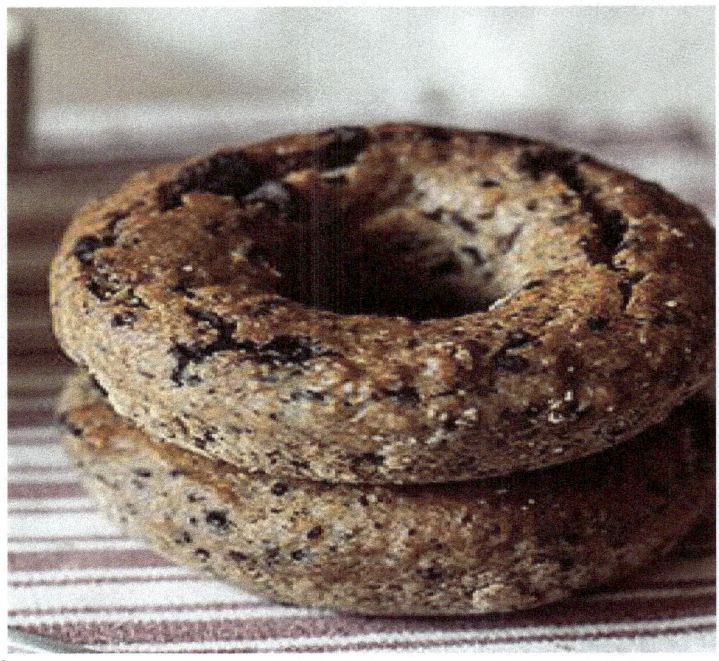

Ingredients

- 200 g type 0 flour
- 20 g corn starch
- 1 sachet of natural yeast for sweets
- 100 g of coconut flour
- 100 g of corn oil
- 100 g of velvety tofu
- 150 g of maple syrup (or agave)
- 150 g soy milk (or other vegetable milk)
- 100 g dark chocolate
- 1 pinch of salt
- mint to taste

PREPARATION!

The first steps

- Sift the flour, starch and baking powder into a bowl. Finely chop the mint and dark chocolate, with an immersion blender instead blend the velvety tofu.

We mix

- Now combine the dry ingredients with those in the bowl, then add the chopped coconut flour, chocolate and mint and finally the salt. Stir in order to mix everything well and at this point add the liquid ingredients or the blended tofu, maple syrup, milk and oil. With energy you absorb all the liquids obtaining a fairly liquid compound.

We bake

- Oil and flour some donut molds. Pour in the mixture just obtained and bake at 180 degrees for 30 minutes. Let cool to room temperature before serving.

48. **WHOLEMEAL PUMPKIN PIE**

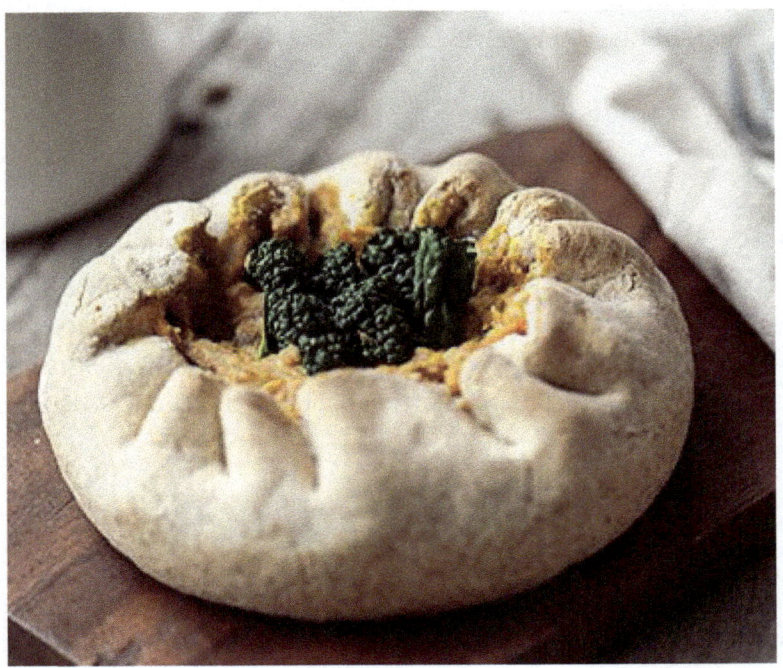

Ingredients

For the pastry

- 150 g of flour 0
- 150 g of wholemeal spelled flour
- 130 g of lukewarm water
- 13 g of brewer's yeast
- g of salt
- tablespoons of extra virgin olive oil

For the filling:

- 1 clove of garlic

- 200 g of boiled pumpkin pulp
- 100 g of boiled potatoes
- 20 g of porcini mushrooms
- tablespoons of sesame
- fresh or powdered ginger
- extra virgin olive oil
- salt and pepper
- Tools: blender or food processor, for cake mold salt of 26 cm

PREPARATION!

We prepare the wholemeal shortcrust pastry

- Sift the two flours and mix them with the brewer's yeast previously dissolved in half the warm water. Add the oil and salt and continue to work everything with your hands slowly adding the rest of the water. As soon as you have obtained a homogeneous dough, knead it for another 5 minutes and then let it rise at about 28 degrees for about 1 hour covered with a damp cloth.

The stuffing

- Leave the porcini mushrooms to soak for about 30 minutes. In a non-stick pan, heat a drizzle of extra virgin olive oil and sauté the garlic with the mushrooms that you have drained and coarsely chopped. Separately, blend the pumpkin pulp and the boiled potatoes, then add the porcini mushrooms without garlic, sesame seeds, ginger, salt and pepper.

Ready for the oven

- Roll out the thin dough a few millimeters thick and line a cake mold. The thinner it will be, the less thick it will be once cooked. Prick the pastry on the base and fill it with the pumpkin cream. Bake at 190 ° C for 35/40 minutes.

49. VEGAN PEAR, CHOCOLATE AND APPLE PIE

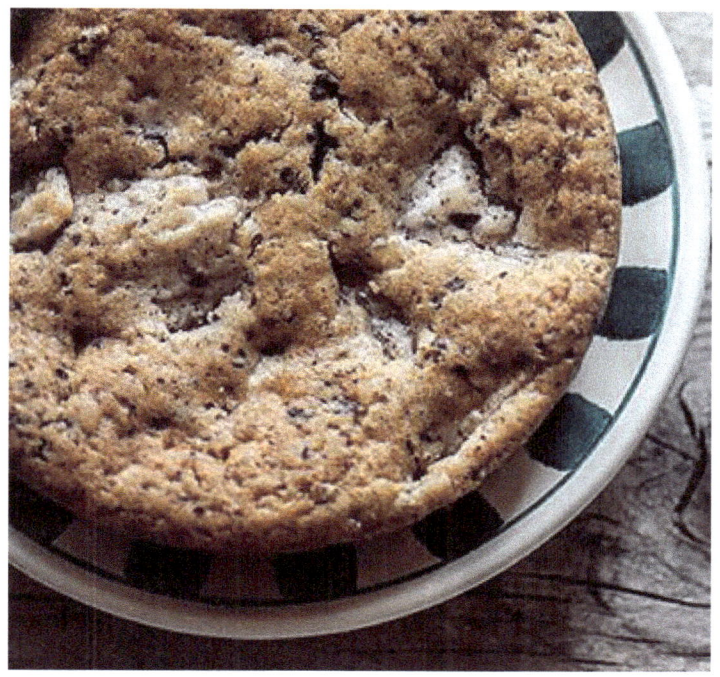

Ingredients

- 100 g of type 0 flour
- 200 g of type 2 flour (semi-wholemeal)
- 150 g of brown sugar
- 250 g of soy milk
- 110 g of corn oil
- 400 g of pears and apples
- 100 g of dark chocolate
- 1 sachet of cream of tartar based yeast (16 g)
- a pinch of salt

PREPARATION!

- In a large bowl, sift and then mix the dry ingredients, then the flour, yeast and sugar to remove any lumps present. Chop the dark chocolate with the blade of a knife, I recommend choosing one with a good percentage of cocoa, at least 75%. On the other hand, coarsely chop the fruit in a small bowl. If you have bought organic, you can also keep the peel.

We mix

- Add the salt to the flour and, slowly, the liquid ingredients. Continue to mix, adding the apples and pears cut into small pieces until the mixture is homogeneous and fairly liquid.

In the oven

- Grease an opening circle pan with flour, pour all the dough into it and bake at 175 degrees for 40 minutes. Let cool and serve lukewarm.

50. VEGAN MUFFINS WITH ZUCCHINI AND DRIED TOMATOES

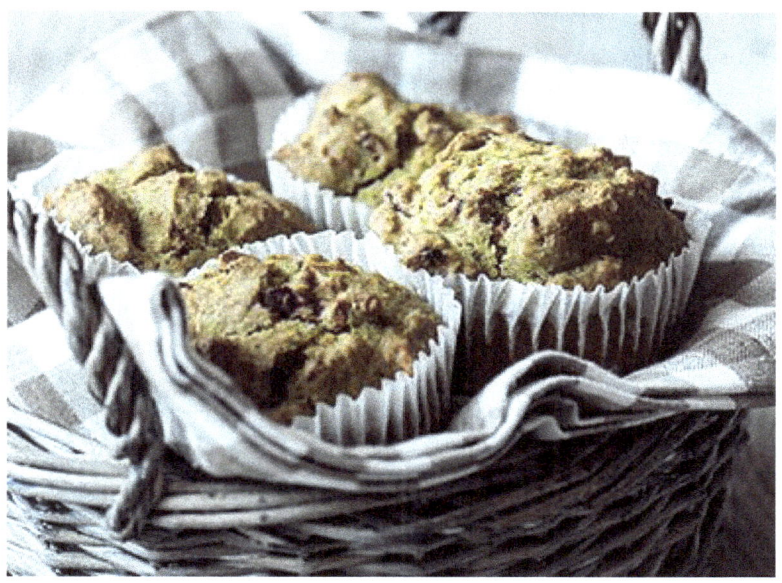

Ingredients

- 200 g of 0 or wholemeal flour
- 8 g of yeast for savory preparations or cream of tartar
- 30 g of potato starch
- 50 g of extra virgin olive oil
- 300 g of zucchini
- 6 g of salt
- 50 g of almonds
- 30 g of dried tomatoes

PREPARATION!

Preparations

- Soak the dried tomatoes for about 30 minutes in warm water. Alternatively, you can also use semi-dried tomatoes, taking into account that they contain a fair amount of preservation oil. Then chop the almonds finely and, with the help of a grater, the courgettes a little more coarsely.

We combine the ingredients

- In a bowl, sift the flour, baking powder and starch. This operation is very important to have a product that, after cooking, is softer and easier to digest. Now add the other ingredients and then the extra virgin olive oil, salt, courgettes, almonds and tomatoes that you have chopped separately after squeezing them from the soaking water.

Let's mix and ... in the oven!

- Mix the ingredients vigorously in order to obtain a very homogeneous mixture. If the dough is too dry you can add some soy milk and make the mixture more manageable. Fill muffin cups and bake at 180 ° C, static oven, for about 20 minutes. With a wooden snack towards the end of cooking, check that once inserted and extracted it is not moist. Let cool and serve (even lukewarm).

Recipe

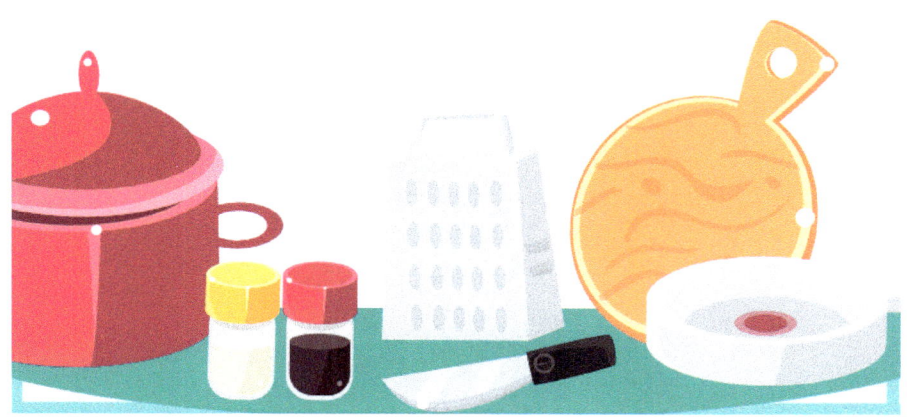

Lightning Source UK Ltd.
Milton Keynes UK
UKHW020721270521
384465UK00005B/114